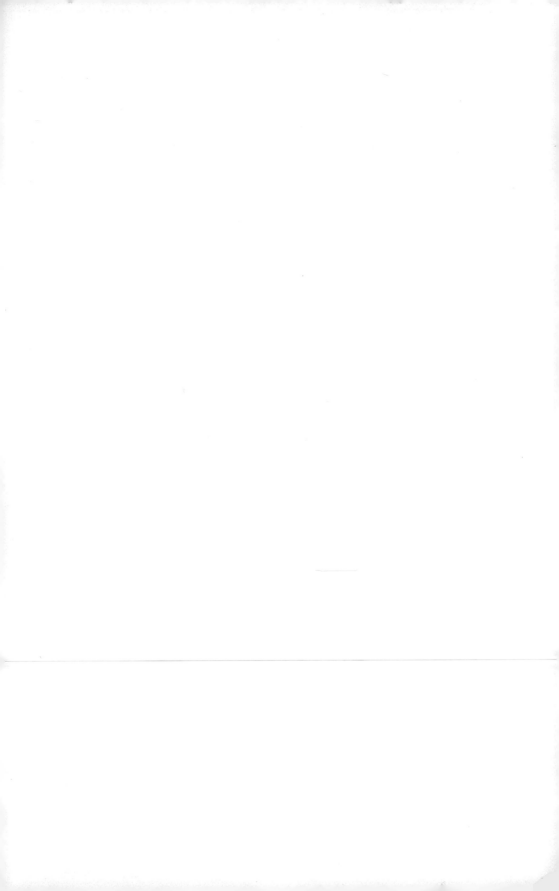

Community Services for the Mentally Retarded

Community Services for the Mentally Retarded

ARNOLD BIRENBAUM, Ph.D.
Professor of Sociology
St. John's University

and

HERBERT J. COHEN, M.D.
Professor of Pediatrics and Rehabilitation Medicine
Director of Rose F. Kennedy University Affiliated
Facility
Albert Einstein College of Medicine

Rowman & Allanheld
PUBLISHERS

ROWMAN & ALLANHELD

Published in the United States of America in 1985
by Rowman & Allanheld, Publishers
(A division of Littlefield Adams & Company)
81 Adams Drive, Totowa, New Jersey 07512

Copyright © 1985 by Arnold Birenbaum and Herbert J. Cohen

Library of Congress Cataloging in Publication Data

Birenbaum, Arnold.
Community services for the mentally retarded.

  Bibliography: p.
  Includes index.
   1. Mentally handicapped—Services for—United States.
2. Mentally handicapped—Services for—United States—
Finance. 3 Mentally handicapped—Government policy—
United States. I. Cohen, Herbert Jesse, 1935-
II. Title.
HV3006.A4B5   1984   362.3′83′0973   84-15905
ISBN 0-86598-151-5

84 85 86 / 10 9 8 7 6 5 4 3 2 1

Printed in the United States of America

To our parents
Molly Birenbaum Weiner and Louis Weiner
and
Barnet and Edith Cohen

Contents

Tables and Figures

Preface and Acknowledgments

Spurred by civil rights legislation for the disabled, and funded by the social welfare legislation of a progressive Congress and by a president who sought his place in history in the making of foreign policy, community care for the mentally retarded in the 1970s was a comparatively rosy picture of reasonable proportions. All of the assumptions established during those heady days were swept away in the 1980s by new federal policies which sought to cap entitlements and return social welfare management responsibilities back to the states. Moreover, the states themselves drastically reduced expenditures since their tax revenues shrunk during the Reagan recession.

What does community care mean today in the context of these changing policies and fiscal conditions? First, mental retardation has not changed. It is a lifelong behavioral phenomenon whether its cause is social, psychological, or biological, or in some combination. The impairments associated with this disabilty interfere with learning and with social and physical development, making independent living problematic for many mentally retarded persons. Second, the human and social costs to the population have not changed. One out of every six or seven families is directly affected by this disability; and education, habilitation, and other special programs are far more costly than programs for some other disabilities, and for the nonhandicapped population as well. Third, the meaning of community care has also remained constant. It is an effort to give people a chance to realize their potential, to reduce the anguish and suffering often associated with custodial care, and to permit the mentally retarded to contribute to the commonly shared goals and aspirations of our society.

In the context of the recent campaign waged against big government, it becomes all the more important to take a close look at what community care provides, how it can be orchestrated, and its costs to society. In so doing, the arguments for or against community care can be examined and the human side of the process explored.

We choose to do this by presenting the story of community care for the mentally retarded in a comprehensive way, indicating the extent to which information is required, plans brought forth, and coordination achieved, in order to establish and maintain even a program modest in size; and there are many fiscal and administrative issues to be resolved. Consequently, a correlative aim of this book is to clarify what is at issue. Only in this way can we fully understand what community care means today.

The translation of community service concepts into viable practices requires information, such as a handbook, easily accessible and unencumbered by scholarly citations in the text. We have chosen to provide a set of references at the end of the text, thereby avoiding their intruding on the ongoing development of a theme or argument.

The meaning of mental retardation in our society has changed, even while the handicapping features of the disability remain the same. Some of the institutionalized obstacles to independence for the mildly and moderately retarded have been overcome with the initiation of education and training at earlier ages, and continuing until age twenty-one. Along with academic skills, prevocational experiences and survival skills related to selfcare activities of daily living are stressed, creating a closer fit between the requirements of adult life and expanded opportunities for community living. Vocational training centers have promoted the employment of their graduates as messengers, waiters, waitresses, and clerical workers. When traditional employment is too demanding, sheltered workshop placement has become an alternative.

Most important, the attitudes of parents, siblings, and the public at large have changed. The idea that every person has a right to as normal a life as possible, whether or not his intelligence is within normal limits, has become a widely accepted notion in American society. This right could be viewed either as compensation for the handicapping conditions of, or as special privileges for, the needy. Rather, we see them as conditions for growth in order to fulfill social responsibilities that go along with independence. It behooves us, then, not to talk in terms of *care*; it is more appropriate to speak of *services* fitted to individual needs, thus avoiding blanket characterizations of mentally retarded citizens.

The authors have benefited from close collaboration with a number of planners, advocates, and scholars in the field of mental retardation. In particular, the late Lee Jacobson read, edited, and gave careful criticism on many aspects of this book. The expert advice on programs and funding provided by Jean Elder and William Copeland was always appreciated. Elizabeth Boggs gave us an insider's view of how some of the recent legislation related to community care of the developmentally disabled was constructed and also made many other important comments about the issues discussed in this book. Stanley Herr informed us of the problems in establishing the legal rights of retarded citizens, and Edward Sagarin not only improved our writing through a careful editing, but also demonstrated his sensitivity to yet another minority population in the United States through the questions he raised and his insightful comments.

This support team was put together through a landmark conference sponsored by the President's Committee on Mental Retardation held in Madison, Wisconsin, in 1980. Many other participants beyond those mentioned above made presentations and remarks on the future directions for community services that were used to frame this work. These contributions are listed in the reference section.

Built on case studies previously published in scholarly journals and anthologies, the section on research on community care includes two chapters based on articles coauthored with Mary Ann Re. These studies could not have been completed without her excellent research skills.

These research reports first appeared in the following places, and we wish to thank the publishers for permission to republish them:

"Resettling Retarded Adults in a Community: Almost Four Years Later" *The American Journal of Mental Deficiency* 83 (1979): 323–29. Copyright 1979, the American Association on Mental Deficiency. (With MaryAnn Re.)

"Mutual Aid Support Among Mentally Retarded Adults Living in Apartments." In Allen D. Spiegel, Simon Podair, and Eunice Fiorito, eds, *Rehabilitating People With Disabilities into the Mainstream of Society,* 1981. Copyright Noyes Medical Publications.

"Family Care Providers: Sources of Role Strain and to Management." *Journal of Family Issues* 4 (1983): 633–58. Copyright Sage Publications. (With MaryAnn Re.)

Finally, the authors wish to express their appreciation to Belle Agatstein, Edna Wagner, Phyllis Zummato and, in particular, to Eva Munoz for their assistance.

Introduction: Progress and Discontinuities

The histories of American welfare institutions and policies clearly reveal that the trends in programming for the habilitation and care of mentally retarded people reflect social and political climates as well as the state of the art of the various helping and learned professions. Federal policies of the 1970s were based on the widespread professional opinion that large and isolated institutions stifled the adaptive skills of those who were placed in them. The populations of these facilities, according to projected goals, were to be decanted, spilling out into programs that would promote individual development in less artificial environments. When President Nixon, spurred by the advice of the President's Committee on Mental Retardation, set his deinstitutionalization targets in 1971 of a one-third reduction in the institutional population by 1980, there were approximately 194,000 mentally retarded people residing in public institutions. While this goal has largely been achieved, and deinstitutionalization has continued to be a desired policy, further expansion of community care has been made more difficult. In the past decade, the number of community residential alternatives has significantly increased, and the number of mentally retarded individuals living at home, or who have always lived at home, has grown as well. Even so, the broader goals of community acceptance and participation, both for persons who are retarded and for their families, are being thwarted or displaced; in some cases, goals are not being met because of community resistance, and in some more general ways, by the federal government itself.

This book is a broad survey of trends in community services for the mentally retarded; it describes programs and their consumers; it examines planning, administration, and funding of programs; and the research and evaluation necessary for decision-making is presented. Through this effort, we will shed some light on the following questions:

- What has return to the community meant for people who have lived in institutions most of their lives?

- Do community programs have the capacity to absorb these clients, many of whom are in need of training, homes, and jobs?
- What services are necessary—and is there evidence to suggest that community services are effective—in habilitating and caring for mentally retarded people?
- What are the current and anticipated consequences of new technology on prevention and care?

Answers to these questions require that we carefully describe and analyze the programs, plans, and politics of community care, focusing on the progress and discontinuities in services found in the course of this review.

It is necessary to start with basic concepts and new ways of understanding mental retardation as a handicapping condition. Some of the past practices in providing services for the mentally retarded have obscured the ways in which this population has been assisted by, and considered part of, family and community life. While state institutions, because of their size, give the appearance of caring for all the mentally retarded, the majority of persons with this disability, including the severely handicapped, have always lived in the community.

Although the option of institutionalization has been available for more than a century, the preference of most American families to keep their offspring at home is demonstrated by the lengths to which parents go to avoid placement in custodial facilities. What has been missing, until recently, has been a range of services within communities to make life easier for the families and to help retarded individuals to function better and live more normally. When it is no longer feasible for a mentally retarded person to live at home, families prefer community residential options, homelike in both scale and atmosphere, to the large and isolated institution.

In the past two decades, the educational, residential and vocational alternatives necessary for maintaining mentally retarded citizens in the community have grown rapidly. These programs represent exciting trends in the development and delivery of community services. Spurred on by consumer activism, initially on the part of families and, more recently, through self-advocacy efforts, there has been a heightened public awareness of the needs of the mentally retarded. Complex portrayals in the mass media, including public interest broadcast forums, have made Americans increasingly knowledgeable about and sensitive to both the similarities of the mentally retarded to the rest of the citizenry, and their distinct differences.

Stories of how disability is made manageable in the community have earned the sympathy of the public, particularly where prominent families are concerned. An important source of support and positive recognition for families was the Joseph P. Kennedy family's public acknowledgment of their retarded daughter at a time when few people admitted to having mentally retarded relatives. Subsequently, the late Vice-President and Mrs. Humphrey spoke on national television about their love for their granddaughter with Down's Syndrome.

As a result of these expressions of family acceptance in the early 1960s, the vast majority of parents clearly and emphatically indicated interest in actively seeking services so their children could remain in the community. Despite these encouraging activities, there is still much to be achieved in developing comprehensive community services, no matter what may be the characteristics of the community, its location and lifestyle.

The choice of community care by families in all geographical areas and social classes is buttressed by informal networks of friends and relatives who help in the care of a relative with special needs. The same informal system of mutual aid also has assisted in the implementation of successful foster care programs. Urban housing patterns, surprisingly, have contributed to the development of residential care programs, since the use of apartments for independent living situations, or clusters of apartments for groups of clients, evokes less community resistance than conversion of single family homes to community residences. Furthermore, in transitional big city neighborhoods, a group residence may, in part, have a stabilizing effect and prevent further urban decline.

This new pattern of service delivery needs to be identified, along with problem areas. Briefly detailed here, the trends discussed below are analyzed in subsequent chapters.

Community Residence Development

Making possible the continuum of services required, the development of community residences is one of the important trends of the past decade. In 1970 just over 600 smaller facilities housed about 9,000 people. Recent reports indicate that by 1977, there were more than 5,000 facilities housing more than 60,000 residents. This is a sevenfold increase in the number of residences and a sixfold increase in the number of residents. The most rapid growth is in the controversial, community-based Intermediate Care Facilities for the Mentally Retarded (ICF-MRs).

However hopeful, mere placement in a small facility, redolent with domesticity, guarantees neither the acquisition of self-care skills nor improved social performance. Effective programming depends on such factors as type of staff and their degree of autonomy, staff compensation, and training, including the quality of supervision, the attitudes of personnel, and the type of programs offered. Moreover, large expenditures of funds, high staff-to-resident ratios, and the provision of highly structured therapeutically oriented facilities fail to guarantee that the retarded client will not exhibit maladaptive behavior in the community. This is not to gainsay the successes following the application of behavioral management techniques by staff well qualified in the use of such tools. In short, the variables are quite complex and interactive.

Critical to successful community placement and maintenance is the provision of support services, including sufficient day activity and recreation services to assure both a range and level of opportunities, consistent with a normal rhythm of day and evening activities suitable for clients of varying capacities. The most effective programs utilize an eclectic approach and maximize access to generic services in the community. Residents live, shop, participate in recreational activities, and sometimes work in their community. Their schedules and activities coincide with the life within the community and not with the requirements of an institution.

Fiscal and Administrative Issues

While the nature of services is changing, so have the mechanisms for funding. In fact, very serious concerns have been expressed in many quarters that the current entitlement programs (the enacted means for extending community services) are not directed toward achieving a coordinated service system.

Some of the key fiscal issues and administrative obstacles can be seen as outcomes of the political exchanges between professionals and the representatives of political leaders who wish to contain the extent of government intervention at a time when there is a fiscal crisis at national and state levels. As a result of these critical factors, there are some sharp policy discontinuities:

1. Our national expenditures for mental retardation services are already sizable—close to $14.33 billion in 1983—with an estimated $6.93 billion emanating from the federal budget. At a time when stated federal policy encourages deinstitutionalization, a very sizable and increasing proportion of federal expenditures under the Title 19 Medicaid program is targeted to provide institutional care. States have felt the need to plan expenditures of large sums, projected at close to $1 billion, on capital construction to capture these federal dollars. Most of the funds are targeted for large institutions to enable them to qualify for ICF-MR funding. The rest is used to support medically oriented community service models deemed unsuitable by many professionals.

2. In the last two decades,the enactment of a myriad of federal entitlements has resulted in a tremendous period of growth in the social service and selective medical care programs. Yet, linkages between programs are poor; bureaucratic restrictions are numerous; there is considerable fragmentation; and there is no central authority at a federal level (and none often at other government levels) to reconcile and coordinate the various funding streams. In fact, some federal programs are created and implemented with little or no input from local authorities. Consequently, federal program directors or staff personnel sometimes promulgate extensive, unrealistic, or inappropriate regulations, which the local communities or service providers must attempt to meet.

3. Poorly coordinated services make continuity problematic. A reasonable continuum of care is rarely provided, and rational service systems are the unusual exception. Even where a system exists, it usually lacks flexibility

and is in no way comprehensive in offering a variety of options to those seeking care or treatment.

4. Title 18 (Medicare) and Title 19 (Medicaid) funding have expanded the use of nursing homes for the mentally retarded. An estimated 100,000 retarded individuals reside in these facilities, and it is questionable whether they are receiving adequate care and appropriate programming.

5. With a greater emphasis on community care, there is a need to train prospective employees and professionals to a level of competency so they may more adequately serve the children and adults under their care. Increased emphasis on the interdisciplinary training process can assure a greater coordination among the service personnel and provide for a better understanding of the system on which it depends for much of its support.

The recent pattern of growth is based on funding consumer organizations as direct service providers, including private, for-profit corporations. In consequence, the responsibility for services in some states has shifted from monolithic state systems to an uncoordinated distribution of diverse service providers. The respective roles and responsibilities of the public and private sectors are assessed in a section on service planning, program administration and funding. Accordingly, the following questions are addressed: (a) How can local service providers receive sufficient autonomy and flexibility to pursue client goals while, at the same time, be kept accountable to basic standards of service? (b) Which agencies—federal, state, or local—best assure fiscal accountability, program quality, and accessibility? (c) How can we strike a balance between a publicly financed, but largely privately operated, community residential and/or service system?

Assuring the Viability of Comprehensive Community Services

What follows is a record of how community services have become stabilized, won community support, and are threatened by policies that seek to let loose the forces of the marketplace in social and medical services. At the same time, it should be recognized that we are at the end of the heroic period in the innovation of community concepts of care. The new epoch eschews grand claims; it is based on increasing knowledge and insight on what works and does not work in programming. The third section, on research and evalution of community services, contains a general review of this topic and some selected case studies.

While utopian thoughts have utility,it is now becoming possible to utilize research findings to operationalize such concepts as normalization. More concretely, the comprehensiveness and viability of community care for the mentally retarded may in the future be measurable by valid indicators of quality and effectiveness, moving beyond unrealistic and moralistic pro-grammatic statements.

In this richly complex environment, management needs to know how to use human resources wisely and effectively. Planning must encompass entire human systems; programming for service systems should not only include establishing and obtaining goals for individual clients, but avoiding staff demoralization by including them in decision-making that affects clients. Current wisdom about staffing presents something of a paradox, particularly when services are so intensified that clients are not permitted to be independent. This condition reflects the built-in ambivalence of many human service roles; staff are used to provide care or to act as enablers for clients.

Management also needs to know how individual clients and families are linked to these complex service networks they have organized. In this kind of environment, staff have to be able to team up across agency lines and communicate in conference with each other for the benefit of the client. When staff are selected, the need to possess or acquire these skills should be recognized.

Throughout the 1980s, we need to know how to use resources more wisely and effectively, improve service coordination, and use a greater proportion of funds on direct services. At the same time, we have to learn how to assure that quality services are provided and accountability maintained in decentralized community-based services. This book is dedicated to showing how this can be done and what steps are needed to expand such services to reach everyone in need.

Part One

Programs and Consumers

1

Changing Concepts and Policies

Since the early 1960s, a spate of new ideas in the field of mental retardation has supported a shift of emphasis from institutional to community services. Some of these ideas derive from solid research (usually federally funded); some are still to be proven objectively. Even in the field of community programs, there has been a discernible shift in emphasis from the idea of *care* to the idea of *habilitation*—to educate or train persons who are mentally retarded to function better in society. These new ideas are emerging in response to increased recognition of the adaptive capacities of mentally retarded persons and their families, the knowledge that retarded persons, like all others, can grow and develop in a responsive and self-enhancing environment.

Ideas or concepts are not merely abstractions, but ways of increasing the understanding and control over physical reality and human experience. The development of concepts is an enterprise in which all human beings engage. Over the course of history, human beings have used ideas to solve such practical problems as how to grow more food, move heavy objects, or remove water from a mine shaft. In turn, the solutions to these tasks have been used as models for how other things work. Knowledge of the human body and mind seems to follow such a model. An accurate model of how the heart and circulatory system worked, for example, was not developed until William Harvey used the pump—an invention of his time—as a representation of the functions of the heart.

New words and new meanings speak to us as evidence that the times are changing. The social and political experiences of critical epochs produce new concepts. In turn, these new concepts give us an added understanding of new social relationships, showing us what has been gained and what has been lost through different historical epochs. While not always the recommended treatment, the late nineteenth century witnessed the origins of asylums for those who could not fully care for themselves, and asylums became a dominant principle of public policy. Institutionalization was based on the two notions that have been dispelled in recent decades as a result of the advances in biological and psychological research: that retarded people are "unimprovable" and that heredity is the main cause of their retardation.

The concept of mental retardation has shifted considerably since these ideas dominated the scientific and popular scene. Today it is known that the adaptive capacities of persons labeled mentally retarded can be strengthened. The model of impairment that is being utilized views the retarded person as having developmental needs that must be met for growth to occur.

The experiences of ex-inmates in mental retardation institutions, who either escaped or were released into the community, provided a clue to the inadequacy of prior concepts of mental retardation in guiding the establishment of provisions for mentally retarded persons. In many cases, the former inmates were able to find and hold jobs, marry, and raise families and did not become a special burden to local authorities. In contrast to the dire predictions about their socially pathological behavior, they neither committed more crimes than the rest of the population, nor produced large numbers of severely retarded children. Despite these interesting findings, there are major difficulties in interpreting these studies in the absence of data on the level of functioning of the subjects when they were children, or of knowledge of whether they were in any way representative of the population in residential institutions.

In the pre–World War II era, admission to institutions did not involve meeting specific evaluation criteria from which careful judgments were made about level of functioning. Placement in institutions occurred for many reasons other than clear evidence of severe mental retardation. Some people were judged to be nuisances or troublemakers by families, courts, or influential members of the community; many were orphans or persons for whom no other placement could be found. Some were mentally normal but otherwise handicapped, such as epileptic, blind, or deaf. There is no way of knowing to what extent the followup studies tracked those who should never have been placed in institutions by any standard used today.

The concept of mental retardation that is used today in the human service field recognizes the complexity of this condition and the need for careful diagnosis. The comprehensive definition developed by the American Association on Mental Deficiency includes subnormality in both intellectual skills and social adaptation, occurring prior to age 18:

> Mental retardation refers to significantly subaverage general intellectual functioning existing concurrently with deficits in adaptive behavior, and manifested during the developmental period.

According to this 1977 American Association on Mental Deficiency definition, for the diagnosis of mental retardation there must be both substantial failure in daily activities, or adaptive behavior, and an IQ of less than 70. This definition was established to avoid the bias of testing: children from low-income and minority groups are identified at school age as retarded far out of proportion to their numbers, in comparison to children from more advantaged families or nonminority populations. The use of the IQ test alone as a basis for assignment to special classes has been shown to be affected by cultural bias. Moreover, the mere fact of mental retardation is not justification for placing anyone in a segregated setting.

Recently, experts have argued that what constitutes mental retardation must be seen in relation to the demands that social statuses and roles set for people.

> Mental retardation, as an inclusive concept, is currently defined in *behavioral* terms involving these essential components: *intellectual function*, adaptive behavior and *age of onset*. The causes of retardation are irrelevant to the definition, whether they are organic, genetic or environmental. What is indicated is that at a given time a person is unable to conform to the intellectual and adaptive expectations which society sets for an individual in relation to his peers. In this sense, mental retardation is a reflection of social perception aided by a variety of clinical and nonclinical techniques of identification. [italics in the original.] American Association on Mental Deficiency;

This is not to say that mental retardation is not real; rather, it reflects a limitation in capacity to cope, a limitation more severe in a complex society than in a simple one.

Mental retardation is a condition of major importance to those concerned about public health and education in the United States. The prevalance of this disablity is open to debate, but it is generally considered to be a life-long condition requiring intervention on many levels. Depending on methods of classification and varied estimates, mental retardation affects anywhere from 1 to 3 percent of the total population of the country. Whatever the true prevalence rate, mental retardation is one of the leading disabling conditions in our population.

In the last twenty years, the definitions of who is mentally retarded and to what degree have changed. The revised scales found in Table 1.1 were adopted by the American Association on Mental Deficiency in 1983. Despite the use of intelligence tests to determine different levels of impairment, the professionals in the field strongly support the use of scales based purely on measurements of adaptive behaviors. The levels of mental retardation defined in Table 1.1 are translated into specifications of the prognosis—the degree of independence and achievement (i.e., functioning in school and the community)—in Table 1.2.

The fundamental requirement for establishing services for the mentally retarded is a full understanding not only of how this disablity affects the individual, but also that it has an impact on the family and the community. The life cycle of the retarded individual sometimes meshes with the cyclical character of family life and the dynamics of community institutions, agencies, and opinion. Yet there are critical times when the individual's needs are not synchronized with family and community. Community services for the mentally retarded are built around knowledge of these factors.

A Continuum of Services

The mentally retarded in society are in some ways like other people, and in some ways not. Insofar as most are similar to others as children, they require

Table 1.1   Level of Retardation Indicated by IQ Range Obtained on Measure of General Intellectual Functioning

Term	IQ range for level	(Code)
Mild mental retardation	50–55 to approx. 70	(317.0)
Moderate mental retardation	35–50 to 50–55	(318.0)
Severe mental retardation	20–25 to 35–40	(318.1)
Profound mental retardation	Below 20 or 25	(318.2)
Unspecified		(319.0)

Note: Levels of retardation are identified with the same terms as those used in previous AAMD manuals. The IQ ranges for levels are generally consistent with those suggested by the American Psychiatric Association in their *Diagnostic and Statistical Manual III*, but a narrow band at each end of each level was used to indicate that clinical judgment about all information, including the IQs, and more than one test, the information about intellectual functioning obtained from other sources, etc., is necessary in determining level. Thus, someone whose Full Scale Wechsler IQ of 53 might be diagnosed as either mild or moderate, depending on other factors, such as the relative difference in Performance and Verbal IQ or results of other tests. *Source:*   H. J. Grossman, ed, *Manual on Terminology and Classification in Mental Retardation* (Washington, D.C. American Association of Mental Deficiency, 1973).

the same opportunities to develop and acquire the capacity to create and maintain attachments to others, and to acquire social as well as technical skills and knowledge. Insofar as mentally retarded persons are different from others as children (and as adults), they require more aid in learning the essential skills and in dealing with their social and physical surroundings.

Public policy and the efforts of human services workers in public and private agencies in the 1970s have produced a complex set of community-based services for mentally retarded persons. These services belong in the community because most of those in need of services, whether mildly, moderately, or severely retarded, are found living with their families in natural homes, in homelike domiciles, or in more managed or standardized kinds of residential settings (e.g., Intermediate Care Facilities).

The behavioral and biological sciences are now at the point in the evolution of knowledge of human development where there is more or less agreement on what social and physical preconditions support growth. There is even substantial agreement that mentally retarded persons require three types of services—developmental, supportive, and protective—depending on how much assistance is needed in each case. Some of these services are already found in the human and health service systems, while others are more exclusively for the mentally retarded persons and their families.

Table 1.2 Prognosis and Expected Functional Level, Based on Degree of Retardation

Levels	Academic potential	Activities of daily living (ADL)[a]	Travel capability	Vocational ability
Border-line	Educable, with potential up to about 6th-grade level.	Fully independent	Independent	Employable without special help, though may need vocational training for competitive employment.
Mild	Educable, to 4th- or 5th-grade level (or less). Capable of reading and writing.	Relatively independent in all areas; some training might be required.	May require travel training to use public transportation.	Employable, but often needs some special training if competitive employment is feasible.
Moderate	May read or write, but very limited (1st- or 2nd-grade level).	Trainable for all ADL. Can dress, be toilet trained, prepare food.	Travel only with special training. Usually requires special transport.	No real competitive employment except in restricted setting; sheltered employment likely with specialized training.
Severe	Unlikely to read or write.	Partially trainable. Should acquire most ADL skills. Is toilet trainable, can dress, but may require assistance.	Very limited independent travel potential.	Sheltered employment only, special training required.
Profound	None	May sometimes be toilet trained and dress with assistance. In general, very dependent.	May or may not be ambulatory. Requires special transport.	Very limited trainability for vocational functions.

[a] Dressing, feeding, bathing, routine self-care, toileting.

Source: Adapted from H. J. Cohen, "Introduction," *Pediatric Annals* 11, no. 5 (May 1982).

DEVELOPMENTAL SERVICES

Every individual requires an appropriate environment for growth. This begins with prenatal care, postnatal child and maternal care, and assessments of growth and development. All citizens should have access to these services. Health services are particularly important for mentally retarded persons, to limit the impact of their associated impairments. Access to general health services can reduce the number of days lost from illness in preschool and school programs.

Early childhood identification and intervention programs for retarded children are designed, first, to determine who has developmental problems and to instruct or encourage families to interact effectively with children at risk. These programs teach parents how to stimulate and teach their children if the child's ability to learn is limited. The impaired child must be met more than halfway in areas where the normal child will learn spontaneously by imitation of others.

Education for all children has become a public responsibility. Children are to be placed in the "least restrictive environment" so they can more easily acquire personal care and cognitive skills through association with normal peers. While there is great debate over the merits of "mainstreaming" handicapped with other children, many school districts provide a variety of opportunities for both groups to mingle to a greater or lesser extent.

Recreational and physical activities promote the development of social skills, fitness, coordination, and a sense of achievement. Programs designed for retarded persons at any age can expand the range of the individual's activities and eliminate a sense of isolation. Sports or athletic events are also often a fulfilling lifetime interest.

Work is a central life interest for most Americans. Vocational training is necessary to take advantage of the individuals' strong motivation to utilize their potential productively. It is also important to be aware of the consequences of the stigma of specialized vocational training programs for mildly retarded persons seeking to pass or meld into the general population. Vocational training programs are available for persons at various levels of skill, from those who can find and keep a job in competition with others in the labor market, to those who will remain in sheltered settings and occupational day centers. Recent research confirms the tentative findings of two decades ago that some persons classified as severely retarded can be productive in an economic sense when properly trained and placed in a supportive environment.

SUPPORTIVE SERVICES

To take advantage of attained skills, families and individuals may sometimes have to receive help to sustain independence. Evaluation and counseling services are viewed as a first line of inquiry, assessing the need for support services in collaboration with the client and family.

Services are frequently required to help a family with the care of a retarded person. Respite services, for example, allow a family to take a break from the demanding routine of nurturing a mentally retarded child. Helping to prepare an adult to move into a group home or other residential option may involve intervention by a case worker, who may assist the family in giving up its total involvement with or overprotection of the retarded adult, as much as he helps that person make the transition to a new home.

A range of residential living programs have been established in many communities, and client goals vary from setting to setting. A mild or moderately retarded adult, for example, can live in his or her own home, be involved in competitive employment or vocational activity, and receive little or no support services. Providers of family care may merely create a normal living environment or teach activities of daily living to a moderately or severely retarded child or adult. Moderate or mildly retarded adults in such settings are at times involved in competitive employment or vocational activity, and merely require refinements of activities of daily living skills to enable them to move into a group home or live independently at some later date. Employment encompasses a variety of work activities and settings. Adults often need assistance in finding jobs and learning how to keep them. Less able adults may require work activity in noncompetitive situations.

Intermediate Care Facilities for the Mentally Retarded (ICF-MRs) involve supervised living and programmatic arrangements for groups of persons and provide highly structured services. The staff generally emphasizes activities of daily living, the elimination of problem behaviors, or the participation in vocational activities. Larger institutions have been converted into ICF-MRs, while smaller units (with a capacity of fifteen or less) for the mentally retarded are increasingly found in the community, particularly as funding mechanisms encourage their growth, often as conversions from larger group residences to become eligible for federal reimbursement for residential care.

Mobility and transportation are necessary for individuals who are to participate in community life. A range of aids may be necessary, some of which enhance a handicapped person's capacity to get around on his or her own using mass transportation, while others involve special minibuses or jitneys.

Like others, a retarded person has a need to feel close to others, yet often he finds it difficult to establish friendships because of limited communication skills or lack of self-confidence. These inherent difficulties are aggravated by frequent residential placements. Sometimes the mentally retarded seek the intimacy of marriage and family life. Counseling is helpful in drawing out the person's wants, needs, and capacities to sustain this type of relationship. Ranges of alternatives are available under the general title of family, only some of which involve having and raising children. There are also many questions concerning sexuality in which retarded persons require counseling.

Finally, the processes of maturation and aging require counseling, and perhaps medical intervention for the mentally retarded, to help the individuals deal with declining physical functions.

PROTECTIVE SERVICES

Normal living involves some risks as well as some built-in protections (e.g., fire codes). The retarded individual, depending on the nature of the deficits and concomitant handicaps, may need additional protective services. Conversely, overprotection discourages normal living: development requires opportunities to learn, to achieve, and to take some risks. Yet the absence of all protection against injury or loss of life does not guarantee successful adaptation. A careful assessment must be made for each retarded person as to the type of protection required. At a minimum, our society can safeguard the rights of retarded persons and protect them from harm. Although there is a growing and encouraging movement toward self-advocacy on the part of the mentally retarded, legal guardianship and conservatorship are needed to represent the interests of those more severely impaired individuals who cannot protect their own self interest. Such a court-appointed person should, first and foremost, strive to enhance the individual's rights to decision-making (guardian of person) and, second, provide assistance in managing assets, if any. Guardian counseling and advocacy can be provided through a personal representative, an individual chosen by or for the retarded person where legal guardianship is not needed. This service is especially useful in dealing with developmental and supportive service systems. In short, the retarded person is guaranteed the same equal protection and due process of law available to all citizens under the constitution by having someone to assist in asserting his or her rights.

Those who are vulnerable to exploitation need protection against abuse and neglect. The severely and profoundly retarded share with the elderly a need to be protected from some "caretakers." Retarded persons also may need protection in employment situations to avoid unfair exploitation, to receive fair compensation according to ability, and to assert their right to work. Work incentives should be available to retarded persons, despite the fact that they are not always able to achieve a high level of productivity.

Service Providers

The new approach to the delivery of human services must include a discussion of who does what in order to habilitate, remediate, and ensure maximum growth for persons with intellectual and adaptive deficits that are discovered early in life. The lines of demarcation in this field are blurred between health, education, and human service providers. Many newly conceived tasks may be performed by members of various occupational and professional groups. But no matter which professionals provide the services, their salaries, wages, and fringe benefits comprise an enormous part of the costs of community services for retarded persons. It is conservatively estimated that 70 percent of the expenditures for the mentally retarded in the United States are for personnel.

Two types of activities and roles assist the mentally retarded in the community. *Direct service* involves what is considered "active treatment," generated by educators, psychologists, social workers, speech therapists, vocational rehabilitation counselors, occupational therapists, residential care specialists, recreational therapists, nurses, and physicians. *Indirect service* is provided by those who coordinate and speak up for the retarded person and, when necessary, with his natural or foster family. New roles have been created for people who are called public advocates, personal representatives, and case managers. Community-oriented services have permitted a variety of professionals, such as psychologists or social workers with extensive academic training and practical experience, to become case managers and chief executive officers. Case managers coordinate the complex array of services needed by one individual; executive officers assure the availability to all of the required elements in the array. The new title of Qualified Mental Retardation Professional to designate a current service role is being used by certifying commissions and state regulatory agencies who set standards for the performance of service coordinative functions in the residential and day programs established in the community.

Two facts about services to mentally retarded persons must be understood in consideration of the adequacy of existing programs. First, there is immense variation in the types and levels of services required by an individual, depending on his intellectual and adaptive functioning. Many mentally retarded persons are able to work and meet their own basic living costs, and either do not require special assistance or require it at infrequent intervals. Other mentally retarded persons, in contrast, are severely dependent and require 24-hour-a-day care or supervision; in extreme cases, they may need to be fed and bathed. In between these extremes fall the persons who, because of their level of mental retardation, require one or more of a variety of combinations of housing and services. Second, the types of services that are needed by a particular mentally retarded person will vary over a lifetime. As the individual develops and goes through the life cycle, his needs will change.

A look at community residential services will help us understand the importance of these considerations.

2

Varieties of Living Experiences

A man in his early thirties lives in a large city. At seven A.M. the alarm rings in his room. His roommate has long since gone to work. After turning off the alarm, he gets out of bed, washes, shaves, brushes his teeth, and has his breakfast. He gets his sandwich for lunch and meets a fellow worker with whom he travels by bus to his shop. At the end of the work day they return home together. Later with his dinner companions, he discusses the events of the day and his plans for the weekend. After dinner, he watches television, has a snack, and talks to a friend about the program on the TV screen. After saying goodnight, he goes off to his room where he finds his roommate already asleep. Tomorrow, he thinks, they will have to clean up their room. He turns on the radio very softly, so as not to disturb his roommate, in order to relax before going to sleep. He sets his alarm so that he will wake up at seven o'clock and be able to arrive at work at the required time. Tomorrow is payday and he thinks about what he will do with the money. Perhaps he will go to the new *Star Wars* movie at the local theater. [Birenbaum and Sirffer 1976.]

Written by one of the authors in 1976, and slightly updated for the 1980s, this passage was an introduction to a longitudinal or prospective study of the resettlement of mentally retarded adults at a privately operated 70 bed community residential facility. This composite picture of a day in the life of an ordinary person is not very astonishing. It is a life of normal appearances and conventional activities. Nothing much happens during this typical day, but less than two years prior to resettlement this mentally retarded adult was housed in a traditional institution in a rural area, a place where he had lived since the age of sixteen. At the state school, as it was known, he spent much of his time waiting for meals, watching television, or wielding a mop in the dormitory which he shared with seventy-nine other men. Despite an IQ of 51 and after eighteen years of institutional living, this man is living in the community, where, with some help, he is utilizing community resources for vocational rehabilitation, recreation and health services.

A composite picture of the deinstitutionalized individual is intriguing but obscures two salient facts about community living. First, the label "mentally retarded" applies to a vast range of handicapped, who require a wide range and type of services. Some mentally retarded persons have achieved independence to such an extent that they are not only independently capable, but even sensitive to the label; they do not wish to be identified as mentally retarded through contact with a specialized agency. Other mentally retarded persons, in contrast, are so multiply handicapped as to be totaly dependent and to require 24-hour care.

In between these extremes are found many mentally retarded persons who require a unique combination of shelter and support services of a less intensive kind. The wide variation of needed services depends on the the client's adaptive skills, age, life experience, and physical and emotional conditions. It would be a simple matter to devise programs for community living if all mentally retarded persons were composites of easily defined characteristics.

Further, the combination of required community services varies over the lifetime of a mentally retarded person. It has not always been obvious that changes occur as mentally retarded persons move through the life cycle from infancy to school age to adulthood and, finally, into old age. More important, the process of learning ordinarily acquired in early childhood may in the retarded person extend well into adulthood. As they develop they may require different living experiences, progressing, for example, from group homes to independent living situations. Table 2.1 provides a picture of the variety of residential service models available and describes the clients that can be accommodated in each type of setting, its aims, support services, and staffing.

More experientially and less programmatically, it is useful to distinguish the following general types of residential facilities and levels of service:

- Apartments and homes in which the need for oversight is infrequent, perhaps involving a social worker who visits once a week and is available for emergencies. Supplementary housekeeping services may be required.
- Residences in which there is a need for daily, but not constant, 24-hour supervision, e.g., the supervision may not always be provided on the premises. Perhaps a case manager visits or counseling is provided through a sheltered workshop or in a day activities center. [Several models of 24-hour facilities must be distinguished: a, those in which the staff of the facility is responsible for all "active treatment" on and off the premises; b, those whose residents require nighttime aid, including "awake" and "on duty" staff; and c, those in which one or neither is included.]
- Foster care and living with relatives where the need for either internal (on site) or external supervision may vary from slight to extensive.

The language and concepts of human services often avoid the obvious. Perhaps the most extensive type of developmental, supportive, and protective services for the mentally retarded are the result of love and obligation. Certainly for young mentally retarded persons, the natural family continues to be the major source of care. More than 95 percent of the

Table 2.1 Residential Services Models

Model	Type of setting	Client characteristics (Relate to level of functioning, not to IQ tests)	Program		
			Emphasis	Support services delivery mode	Residential staffing[b]
Independent Living	Own home	Adults, mildly to moderately retarded	Competitive employment Retirement Vocational activities	External Generic	None
Natural home	Parents' home, adaptive parents' home	Children, mildly to profoundly retarded, medically complex, behavior problem	Early intervention Education/stimulation Parent training, as needed Medical/Nursing, Therapies, PR services	Primarily external generic	None
Semi-independent living	CLA minimal supervision Family care homes	Adults, mildly to severely retarded	Self-management Retirement Vocational activities Competitive employment	External Generic	As required at intervals
Supportive living	Group living facility with programming provided and by communicating agencies; 3-bed or	Adults or children mildly to profoundly retarded	Refinement of activities of daily living skills Vocational activities Competitive	External Generic	24 hours or whenever client(s) present

Model	Setting	Clients	Programs	Services	Staffing[b]
	less CLA; foster homes and family care homes		employment Early intervention Education (children) Participation in community activities	Internal (time-limited) External generic (on-going)	24 hours or whenever Client(s) present
Highly structured living	ICF/MR, 15-beds or less; CR, 15-beds or less; CLA, 3-beds or less	Adults or children, mildly to profoundly retarded, problem behaviors, and/or medically complex	Acquisition of activities of daily living skills, modify problem behaviors, vocational activities, competitive employment, stimulation, education (children)		
Institutional living	State centers, MR Units, contracted facilities, ICF/MR, 16 beds or more, CR, 16 beds or more	Adults, severely and profoundly retarded, mildly and moderately retarded, problem behavior, medically complex	Same as highly-structured living (may encompass all programs above)	Internal/external, contracted	24-hour

a Physical handicaps (deafness, blindness, ambulation problems, etc.) can be accommodated in *any* model.

b Staffing may vary as clients are prepared to move to the next model.

Note: CLA = Community living apartment

CR = Community residence

ICF/MR = Intermediate care facility for the mentally retarded

PR = Physical rehabilitation

2.6 million mentally retarded under the age of 21 live at home. Families need services and support to live normally; still, they continue to be a source of care in a world that increasingly disvalues the experience of being a family member.

The family has often been assumed to be too fragile or inadequate to provide care for a mentally retarded child. Thirty or forty years ago, professional opinion encouraged parents to place their retarded children in traditional institutions for the good of the child and of the family. Professionals underestimated the capacity of mentally retarded children to develop, and their disability was seen as destructive to family living. Today such advice is rare. This change has contributed to a reduction in the population of our large public residential facilities and an increase in the average age of residents, despite improvements in the physical arrangements of state schools (now commonly called Developmental Centers), as well as improved staffing and training of residents for more independent living.

According to the Scheerenberger survey conducted in 1979, there were 278 public residential facilities in the United States with a total bed capacity of 155,902 and an average daily census of 139,130 (see Figure 2.1). Between 1972 and 1979, there was an overall reduction of 34,000 residents in these facilities. This rate of decrease of the institutional population appears to be continuing in the 1980s. In 1982 Lakin and associates reported that 119,335 mentally retarded individuals were then housed in public residential facilities. Despite this shift in placement policy and some movement out into the community, 19 percent of the state-operated facilities studied in 1979 remained large-sized, housing more than 1,000 residents, with an additional 70 percent housing more than 200 residents each. Seventy-five percent of the remaining residents of large public institutions are severely and profoundly mentally retarded.

Closer to the family is the group home model, a small residence within a neighborhood. This type of arrangement provides either a long-term or transitional supervised living environment, staffed either by house parents who live in or by two or three shifts of personnel. In 1982 these programs were located at 6,302 sites, serving 58,063 mentally retarded people, in every state. Overall, these programs served a population made up of adults (85%) and children (15%).

Size is a distinctive characteristic of the group home. Results of a 1982 telephone survey found that the average number of beds per home was 9.2, and 91 percent were residences of 15 beds or less. In addition, the survey revealed an additional 10,000 mentally retarded persons living in specially licensed family care and independent apartments in the community.

Traditionally, the cost of care in an institution has been a state responsibility; parents were expected to pay part of the cost, based on their financial ability. In the past decade an increased share of the cost has been assumed by the state and federal governments under Medicaid. Many retarded persons have been placed in skilled nursing facilities or in intermediate care facilities other than those established specifically for the

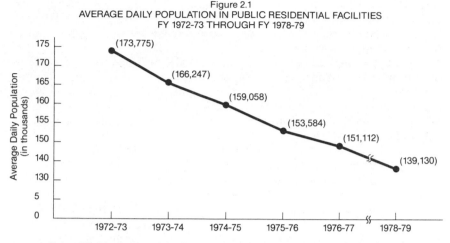

Figure 2.1
AVERAGE DAILY POPULATION IN PUBLIC RESIDENTIAL FACILITIES
FY 1972-73 THROUGH FY 1978-79

Source: R.C. Scheerenberger, *Public Residential Services for the Mentally Retarded,* 1979. National Association of Superintendents of Public Residential Facilities.

mentally retarded. In the 1977 National Nursing Home Survey, it was estimated that almost 80,000, or 6.1 percent, of nursing home residents had a primary or secondary diagnosis of mental retardation. A mentally retarded person is supposed to be placed in a general facility only if it has been determined that this placement is more appropriate than any others, such as a placement in a special intermediate care facility or in a still-less restrictive environment, such as a group home

Many large private as well as public institutions are certified as Intermediate Care Facilities for Mentally Retarded persons. The John F. Kennedy Institute estimates for 1981 show 1,123 ICF-MRs in operation, evenly divided between those with more and those with less than fifteen beds. An ICF-MR is an optional service under Title XIX offered by forty-eight states under their Medicaid programs.

The requirements for an ICF-MR are the absence of need for intensive or skilled nursing and medical services, and the need for 24-hour care with habilitation or rehabilitation. Thus, an ICF-MR is an organization that attempts to provide regular health-related services to a population that can do without skilled nursing or hospital services. While a 24-hour-a-day program of "active treatment" is required, an ICF-MR is not intended to be "medical" in design. Medicaid funds can be used to meet the cost of board and lodging and protective care as well as for meeting the habilitative goals established for residents through individualized programming that constitutes "active treatment." Public facilities are eligible for reimbursement provided that the mentally retarded resident meets the means test and receives active treatment. This financial boost to public institutions was designed to improve services; it has indeed given new life to large and isolated facilities in an age of deinstitutionalization, but it has also contributed to their depopulation as a result of its requirement for more physical space per resident. Whether public or private, "large" ICF-MR facilities are defined has having sixteen or more beds with no upper limit on the total number of beds.

Funding for small public and private ICF-MR facilities have been a state option since 1972. The specific provisions exempting certain small facilities from complying with the institutional life safety codes were included in the regulations several years after certification for larger facilities was begun. While using more flexible physical standards and safety codes for residents who are at least mobile and capable of self-preservation, the small facilities designated as ICFs-MR are still required to provide active treatment. Staffing patterns in small facilities are less comprehensive, because the resident population will be less varied than at larger facilities and will need more outside services.

The development of small facilities, whether certified as ICF-MRs or not, represents another trend in programming. Typically, many essential services for residents are provided in locations other than the residential facility. Bruininks has established in a national survey (1983) that more than 80 percent of all residents in all small community residential facilities, whether designated ICF-MRs or otherwise, leave the facility during the day to receive services in the community or to go to work.

One reason that the variability of the client population of small facilities is less than at large facilities is because of efforts to relax institutional safety standards for small units occupying ordinary housing. The selection process for clients in small facilities is intended to exclude persons deemed incapable of following directions and/or taking appropriate action for self-preservation under emergency conditions, thus excluding nonmobile residents. For this reason placement is often based on regulations directed to protecting life and avoiding injury, rather than on program needs.

It is estimated that only 22 percent of the residents of small public facilities are severely or profoundly retarded, whereas about 42 percent of the residents of small private ICF-MRs fall into this category. Furthermore, the percentage of ambulatory, or nonambulatory but mobile, clients in small facilities is higher than in the large facilities.

Active Treatment

The idea of active treatment provides a way for dealing with complex service requirements of a varied population. Recognizing this complexity, the amendments to the Social Security Act that made the ICF-MR program possible called for the "regular independent professional review of patients," ensuring that individuals would receive the level and type of service they need in the most appropriate setting. Qualified personnel must be involved in programming to see that active treatment takes place and the stated objectives of the institution are achieved.

Active treatment is defined as the development and implementation of an individualized plan to care for clients and direct their participation in professionally developed and supervised activities, experiences, and therapies. An individualized plan sets forth measurable goals and objectives stated in terms of desirable behavior necessary to reach them. The overall purpose of the plan is to help the individual function at the greatest level of independence that he can presently or potentially achieve. The plan is expected to include proposals for moving the client into a less restrictive setting.

Active treatment is a concept that is linked not to location, but to the individual. In other words, block programming, which was the prime mode of the traditional institution, is to be replaced by professionally established developmental goals and support services for each individual. To be certified, a large ICF-MR with a heterogeneous population must provide a full range of rehabilitation specialists. Greater flexibility in staffing is shown toward the small facility. Professional services may be provided by independent contractors (agencies or practitioners) rather than by employed staff, as long as the quality of the provider is assured in the most cost-effective manner. When no resident of a facility requires a particular service, such as physical therapy, that service need not be provided. Similarly, other on-site services, such as nursing, do not have to be present if a physician certifies that the residents do not require it. Finally, staff size at small facilities may be reduced proportionately if residents are scheduled to leave for active treatment elsewhere during the day.

Active treatment involves coordination of all services received, including those inside and outside the facility. This principle is expected to be more than a mere platitude. All individuals who interact with the client are expected to be consistent in encouraging the acquisition of skills. Thus, formal teaching should be reinforced in everyday life by resident living staff, making learning transsituational. For example, a person lives in a small residential facility and goes to an activities day center where an occupational therapist teaches self-feeding skills at lunch. Optimally, the occupational therapist also instructs the staff of the residence how to teach the same skills, so the self-feeding training techniques are practiced at both locations. Staff of the ICF are ultimately responsible for assuring that this coordination among component providers actually occurs.

The ICF-MR is responsible for providing the services that the client requires. The level of funding is far in excess of Supplemental Security Income support for the disabled. If the individuals do not need the comprehensive developmental habilitation, they are not eligible for ICF-MR placement. Alternately, if a facility is incapable of providing active treatment, it cannot be certified as an ICF-MR or be eligible for Medicaid as an inpatient service. The intent of the active treatment regulation is clear. Both utilization review and independent professional review functions are required to ensure that clients are receiving the appropriate services.

The Question of Size

During the halcyon days of normalization, the big facility was universally considered the bad facility. Programming of the type recommended by the concept of active treatment was always considered impossible in large public or private institutions. Certainly one could convincingly argue that size-,combined with a custodial ideology, would lead many managers of these institutions to be concerned with the operations of the domiciliary components, rather than the client's developmental and supportive needs.

Size has another dimension in addition to number of beds. Large traditional institutions are, for the most part, located in rural areas, making access difficult to urban-based outside services. In addition, the distant locations often discourage visits by city families, volunteers, and others who could perform personal representative functions that would ensure the presence of active treatment. Somewhat intimidating, but physically proximate, are large public or private facilities for residential living in densely populated areas.

Identical residential schools in the private sector seldom exceed 500, but hardly qualify as an ordinary way to live. What factors are critical? In a recent study of social behavior inside facilities that varied in size from six to twenty beds, smaller facilities did not encourage greater interaction between staff and residents than larger units. Contrary to current professional wisdom, within that range there was more client-client interaction in larger units than in small ones. These results must be interpreted cautiously, since other desirable behavior, such as acquisition of self care-skills, may correlate differently.

While proponents of normalization may be partial to small facilities, the early trends in ICF-MRs have been toward large private institutions and a renovation of the similarly defined, but somewhat scaled-down public facilities that now meet the Medicaid standards. A number of factors in the process of starting up small ICF-MRs have discouraged their development. First, the modified standards making them feasible were approved for federal reimbursement more than three years after larger facilities were eligible for reimbursement. Second, large private facilities may be cheaper to operate on a per capita basis than small private or public facilities, perhaps because of more efficient use of professional staff and cost effective purchasing practices. Nevertheless, some would argue that additional capital and upkeep costs actually make large facilities more expensive in the long run. An extensive correlation study by Wieck illustrates the multifactorial character of costing issues. Third, providers of small private facilities are often drawn from the voluntary sector, mainly from nonprofit agencies not familiar with medically oriented service standards of the various certifying agencies. For example, voluntary associations wishing to sponsor small ICF-MRs are often discouraged by lengthy delays in receiving Certificate of Need review and approval from the state health systems agencies. These reviews were introduced to limit health care costs by stopping the uncontrolled growth of acute care hospitals. To qualify for placement, clients are required to receive an initial nonreimbursable diagnosis and evaluation at a cost that some nonprofit agencies cannot afford. From the perspective of the manager of a small facility, even more wasteful is the physician recertification of clients' needs (a reimbursable procedure) every sixty days, even when the basic condition does not change. While many of these requirements are paid for by Medicaid, the administrator of a small ICF-MR must contract for them, leaving less time to devote to program planning and active treatment. Fourth, some states have not waived the institutional Life Safety/Fire Safety codes for small facilities that house mobile, nonambulatory clients capable of self-preservation. Similarly, it is costly to implement physical accessibility requirements. These requirements, which call for such arrangements as wide hallways and parking lots, detract from the unobtrusive design of a building and make it all too obvious that an institution of some type, however small, is present.

While small ICF-MRs provide only a tiny proportion of community residential services for the mentally retarded, their numbers have rapidly grown, particulary where the governmental climate has been favorable to them. States which have encouraged the growth of small ICF-MRs through public policy and the allocation of resources have succeeded in overcoming the obstacles involved in obtaining needed approvals. Minnesota, in 1980, funded 194 small ICF-MRs by providing direct technical assistance to potential providers under a federally funded project. This project gave advice and training to small providers at a time when other states in the country had little experience in developing such facilities. The technical assistance team acted as a resource on all issues concerning development, financing, certification, and licensing. Current estimates are that there are now about 1,100 certified ICF-MRs, both public and private. Thus, the ICF-MR model accounts for only about 10 to 15 percent of the community residences or similar living arrangements that have come into being in the last decade.

As the preceding description has emphasized, the development of the small ICF-MRs in the community has taken place where states are most aggressive in seeking federal reimbursement for the costs of this type of residential service. Some observers have argued that these funding mechanisms change the nature of the objectives of community residential services; the origin of the community residential model was based on ideological and physical grounds. Many argue that fiscal factors should not have become the primary considerations, and this has provoked conflict. Proponents of community care have protested that the "medical model" foisted on them by the ICF-MR regulations requires medical certification and participation in treatment planning and implementation. Since the ICF-MR program was an outgrowth of a medically oriented reimbursement mechanism (Title XIX), the requirements are understandable. Still, some consumer and advocacy groups continue to resent the imposition of medical requirements for community residences seeking to maintain conventional living environments. Habilitation, they argue, is not medical treatment. These groups remain unhappy with the growth of the ICF-MR program as the major source of reimbursement for community-based residential care.

Residential care is only one part of the spectrum of community services. In Chapter 3 we discuss the full range of programs necessary for maintaining the quality of life for mentally retarded persons in the community.

3

The Spectrum of Community Services

In the heat created by the recent debate over deinstitutionalization, it is easy to forget that community services for the mentally retarded are nothing new. The first special education classes for mentally retarded children were established more than eighty years ago in Providence, Rhode Island. More than thirty years ago, local and state chapters of the Association for Retarded Citizens initiated school programs for children deemed ineligible for public education. These parent-run associations also began the first sheltered workshops and vocational training programs for the mentally retarded and developmentally disabled when their children were no longer served by school programs.

Families remain the first source of developmental, protective, and supportive services for mentally retarded children. They are also an appropriate part of the network that sustains adults who may have left home. Since they are subject to stress when one of the members is disabled, the family also requires assistance. Most families must also cope with a complex social environment. The modern urban environment, notwithstanding all that social critics say about it, can be made to extend positive opportunities to learn and thrive to all citizens. The problems and potentials in the rural areas are different. For many, the County Extension Service of the Department of Agriculture and the visiting public health nurse service offer the only help available to farm families with handicapped children for whom few group programs exist.

In both settings, rural and urban, prevention programs are needed, in which the stress is on (a) satisfactory prenatal care, (b) constructive approaches to adolescent pregnancies, birth control, and genetic counseling, (c) reduction of alcohol and drugs during pregnancy, (d) efforts to minimize child abuse, (e) conscientious efforts to remove toxins such as lead from the child's environment, (f) accident avoidance (particularly falls and automobile injuries), and (g) the early identification and treatment of disabilities.

Early Intervention

THE FAMILY

The family is a socially flexible unit that can survive the tragedy of disability. Yet the stresses of modern living are such that even the wealthy find it difficult to care for mentally retarded members at home without supportive services. Supplemental Security Income payments, if the family is eligible, are in many cases inadequate to cover the extraordinary costs of care and the related service requirements for low-income disabled children who live with their natural families. Middle-income families not eligible for Medicaid may find that special therapies are not covered by standard health insurance coverage and hence are exorbitantly expensive; yet the child placed out of home could be eligible for this care at greater total expense. As an economic as well as a morally preferred option, the natural family is a far less expensive alternative than government funded residential care.

The financial strains of modern living are matched by the social pressure to lead a normal life by all children in the family. The presence of a mentally retarded child calls into question the family's capacity to engage in the variety of activities that make up a normal life. At times the family with a disabled member needs to get away from the daily responsibilities of care, to find what it is like not to be especially burdened, not to be different. Respite services can spell the difference between family survival and failure, between hope and despair.

Even with financial assistance, with access to respite services the family of the mentally retarded person, whether consciously or unconsciously, must determine if the individual needs of the retarded member are being met but at the expense of the total family unit. Moreover, they need to assure that the growth needs of the disabled child are addressed in an environment that enhances the retarded individual's capacity to cope with the wider community. Psychologists have often noted that this effort has to be made in the face of uncertainty, and rarely do professionals recognize and reward parental and sibling competency. Despite the lack of chronological guidelines, the unavailability of peer comparison, and the inadequate signals for growth transmitted by the child, it is hoped that the natural if limited resources available to the mentally retarded child are be developed to the fullest.

When a handicapped child is present, the family may be considered a system in crisis. The presence of a mentally retarded child always affects social interaction, whether the focus is the psychosocial interior of the family or its points of contact with the outside world. A family that attempts to reduce the consequential and episodic nature of living with a mentally retarded child often has to be trained to seek—even demand—the things all its members need. When the stress on family life threatens its integrity, counseling or family therapy may be necessary to help accelerate the emotional learning process for the client and significant others, to help the parents understand that the interior world they have constructed for their children and themselves may be counterproductive. In modeling themselves after parents of normal children, for example, mothers and fathers in the disabled child's later years may reduce their activity on behalf of their offspring at a time which may be the most difficult for the offspring, a time of transition to adulthood in which "differentness" takes on a new connotation.

PRESCHOOL PROGRAMS

It has been noted that low-income populations are overrepresented among the mildly mentally retarded, far in excess of expected frequencies. Consequently, children of the poor are often found not to do as well in school and competitive employment. The introduction of preschool and early intervention programs, a byproduct of the social legislation of the 1960s, has reduced this pattern of failure. Project Head Start was built on the assumption that early education, parental involvement, and the provision of medical and social services could prepare children of low-income parents to do as well in school as their middle class peers. It was expected that this form of intervention would have an enabling effect, and that children exposed to these programs could eventually leave the ranks of the poor through their own efforts. A variety of programs was created, using different curricula, personnel, and learning materials. Although the first evaluations of these efforts showed disappointing results, newer longitudinal studies have established the effectiveness of early intervention programs of the preschool type, using direct measures of children's actual school performance.

While no comparisons are made with middle-class children, in 1976 low-income children who had attended infant and preschool programs in the 1960s had made more progress in meeting academic requirements than those children who did not attend. Statistical comparisons were made between 1,600 subjects and controls in eleven original projects, with children ranging in age from nine to nineteen, in which effectiveness was identified as a significantly lower frequency of placement in special education classes or by being in grade (held back).

Reading the report in the journal *Science* (1980), it is easy to understand why professionals are enthusiastic about early childhood intervention as a form of secondary prevention. In view of these findings, it is hard to understand the lack of progress in expanding early education efforts for high-risk children, even though extraordinary costs are involved. Only fifteen states currently mandate full school or nursery service for the 3-to-5–year age group. For more severely handicapped children, programs beginning in the first year of life have been developed but are not yet widely available.

While the studies cited above applied primarily to children considered to be organically intact but psychosocially at risk, other recent studies have demonstrated the effectiveness of early intervention techniques with children whose central nervous systems are impaired. An important consequence of some of these intervention programs is the parent support and counseling that is offered which, according to the report of the United Cerebral Palsy Association's Collaborative Project, was one of the most valued and helpful elements of the five programs studied in the project.

Schools

If primary and secondary prevention, along with family support services, are the first prerequisites of a system of community services, schools constitute the foundation. It is now possible for handicapped children to receive educational services from the ages of three to twenty-one in almost every state and, in a few states, even from birth. Under federal legislation that requires a school census of the handicapped, state education agencies reported a total of 4,298,327 handicapped children being served in 1982–83, an increase of 66,045 children over the previous school year, and 589,739 more than were reportedly served in 1976–77. Federal grants for the education for the handicapped are now close to one billion dollars, with estimated local expenditures for special education exceeding six billion.

Handicapped children constitute just less than 10 percent of total school enrollment. Approximately one-sixth of the handicapped children served by the school systems of the United States are diagnosed as mentally retarded. In the school year 1982–83, of the 802,264 children designated as mentally retarded, more than one-third attended regular classes; almost half were in separate classes in community schools; and the remainder were in separate school facilities or other educational environments.

Observers of the school system in this country have raised a number of issues about the way in which programs are created for the mentally retarded. One major concern is the cost of special education, which on a per capita basis exceeds educational expenditures for other children. A study conducted by the state of Colorado computed the average excess cost per pupil for various categorical programs. The cost of educating the trainable (moderately) mentally retarded population was estimated at $2,100 per student annually over and beyond the expenditures for the normal child; programs serving the hearing handicapped, visually handicapped, and multiply handicapped were even more costly.

A great deal of controversy surrounds the policies and procedures used to evaluate the eligibility of children and their subsequent placement in classes for the mentally retarded. In the 1977 landmark Pennhurst case in Pennsylvania, the Association for Retarded Citizens demonstrated that many mentally retarded children were being systematically excluded from receiving a public education. Currently, there is a trend away from segregating mildly and moderately retarded pupils in special classes, and a trend toward "mainstreaming" to a greater or lesser degree.

There is also deep concern about classifying children as handicapped when, in actuality, they do not have such limitations. Studies that focus on the potential for cultural or racial bias in standardized tests show that the results of these tests have led to the inappropriate designation of minority children as mentally retarded; these children were regarded as mentally retarded only when in school. Of considerable interest is the change produced when tests of adaptive behavior in one community were introduced to supplement IQ tests; the number identified as mentally retarded dropped 50 percent.

Many mentally retarded and developmentally disabled children who might have been institutionalized a few years ago are now served in community public schools. A major issue for consideration is what kinds of skills are being transmitted, and for what purposes. There is a critical need to increase the vocational and social skill content of the educational programs available so that the capacity for community participation is enhanced. Some mentally retarded pupils can take vocational training courses with other pupils. Work options after graduation would be increased substantially if occupational training was more extensively available in secondary schools. Preparation for vocational training (as well as the world of work) is useful for mentally retarded persons who will later make the transition to competitive or sheltered employment and adult day programs. Crucial to the viability of community services are programs that enhance independent living through training not only for work, but for daily living, cooking, shopping, use of mass transit, banking, and complying with all the modern personal paperwork requirements.

Adult Programs

SHELTERED WORKSHOPS

Sheltered workshops did not originate in the field of mental retardation. First initiated for the blind, sheltered workshops were soon extended to other disabilities, and many handicapped persons were retrained for competitive employment or found work in these programs on a permanent basis. Many workshops began to serve several kinds of handicapped persons at the same time, but not the mentally retarded.

When mentally retarded children in the 1950s were approaching the age at which they were no longer eligible for schooling, their parents sought entry for them in sheltered workshops for the disabled. The mentally retarded were consistently refused admission because the staff members of these agencies felt that they did not know enough about their condition to be of service. Rather than despair, these pioneers underwrote the establishment of similar programs for the mentally retarded.

These efforts to establish vocational rehabilitation programs were supported by funding from federal and state revenues. A major impetus to the development of vocational rehabilitation programs for the mentally retarded started in 1954, when state divisions of vocational rehabilitation were able to subsidize the rehabilitation of mentally disabled persons for the purpose of making them "fit to engage in a remunerative occupation" (P.L.

83-565). Later, P.L. 88-333 made placement in a sheltered workshop a legitimate reason to subsidize a client's training. Currently there are some 156,457 mentally retarded adults being trained or employed in 5,866 Labor Department–certified programs in the United States. These programs have been successful in helping many mentally retarded persons become self-supporting. Tax monies invested in vocational rehabilitation have shown impressive returns.

A few studies indicate that moderately and severely retarded adults, as well as less impaired persons, can learn surprisingly complex vocational tasks. When properly broken down into a series of sequential steps, such jobs as the assembly of a 52-piece cam switch, requiring the use of five different hand tools, have been mastered by moderately and severely retarded individuals in a demonstration workshop in Oregon. Given an approach to training that allocates sufficient time to the design of learning, with carefully organized procedures, relatively complex tasks can be performed by developmentally disabled people with low levels of intelligence.

ADULT DAY PROGRAMS

In 1980 it was estimated that about 105,500 severely handicapped persons were attending adult day programs. These programs focus on providing training in living and social skills, prevocational and recreational activities, and have become long-term service providers for some of the more severely mentally retarded persons living in the community. Not every client remains in programs that teach the activities of daily living for the remainder of his life. Some centers have been able to provide either paid work or rapid placement of selected clients in more work-oriented services. Recent research has shown that a few clients in adult day programs can achieve wage levels considerably above those sometimes achieved in traditional sheltered workshops. Since productivity is highly valued in our society, it is deplorable that adult clients who do not have access to work are spending a great deal of time (up to six hours daily) in trivial activities that are merely time-fillers. In some instances these persons need health-related support services that should be made available to them in conjunction with gainful employment under the recent amendments to the disability provisions of Titles II, XVI, and XIX of the Social Security Act.

Ensuring an Acceptable Quality of Life

MENTAL HEALTH SERVICES

Growing up and living in the community does not eliminate the stresses of family life or choice of vocation. Mere placement in a community residential setting does not insure that the mentally retarded individual will participate in the new living arrangement in a personally satisfying manner. Some fail to connect with those around them. They remain passive, dependent, unmotivated, socially inept, highly anxious, compulsive, ritualistic, depressed, and socially withdrawn; they may be unable to cope with life unless a wide spectrum of community services is available to help them.

The mental health delivery system is incapable of serving the needs of mentally retarded persons with emotional difficulties. At the same time, the mental retardation service network is not designed for meeting the treatment needs of the mentally retarded person with chronic emotional and behavioral difficulties. The major factors contributing to this sorry state include (a) the lack of knowledge about effective intervention procedures, (b) the shortage of mental health and developmental disabilities agency personnel trained to treat emotional and behavioral disorders in the mentally retarded, and (c) the limited interest in and resources among professional personnel and service agencies for providing the intensive and extensive services needed for effective treatment. As a result, many mentally retarded individuals with psychiatric problems do not receive services from either system.

Unquestionably, we need to know more about how to provide mental health services for mentally retarded persons with different levels of cognition and adaptive behavior. Treatment models based on developmental and social learning theories currently appear to hold some promise for understanding and treating the emotional problems of the developmentally disabled. Procedures that might deal effectively with a variety of difficulties involve social skills training and techniques to alter behavior. Moreover, some of these therapeutic techniques can be used by various treatment agents (e.g., vocational counselors) in the natural environments in which retarded clients live and work.

COMPREHENSIVE COMMUNITY SERVICES

The key areas of comprehensive community service, as noted, include family support, education, vocational training, day activities, mental health services, and prevention efforts. It should also include the provision of health services; here, the emphasis is on access to both generic and specialized service providers. The latter include specialized diagnostic and treatment services; these are best supplied by an interdisciplinary team experienced in the complexities of disability.

To be comprehensive, community services must also include recreational facilities and programs, accessible transportation (alone or with travel training) and advocacy services. A spectrum of accessible community-based living facilities would range from independent living facilities to specialized units emphasizing nursing, supportive care and/or habilitation, or rehabilitation. Finally, case management services, which many consider the glue holding the system together, must be in place to help families negotiate the "system" of possible service; case managers coordinate and monitor the system so that a coherent and effective program plan can be evolved and implemented. Physical accessibility is a key requirement, since accessibility to public facilities is an essential component to facilitating more normal social activities in the community.

There is no strong consensus on what constitutes the spectrum of services required in communities of differing size, but the basic elements of a truly comprehensive approach to community services are enumerated in Table 3.1. In summary, only when a spectrum of services and program opportunities is available and reachable by public or specialized transportation, accessible to the handicapped, and physically located within or close to the home community in which the individual resides, will an acceptable quality of community life for the retarded be achieved.

Table 3.1   Components of a community service system

Comprehensive Diagnostic Services

    Medical (all specialties)
    Mental health
    Psychological testing (nondiscriminatory)
    Social services
    Educational evaluation
    Speech and audiological
    Occupational therapy, physical therapy
    Laboratory (including specialized X-ray procedures, electroencephalograms, and
      routine laboratory tests)
    Genetic counseling and diagnostic services

Habilitation and Service Needs

    Medical and Dental Treatment
        General health and dental care
        Access to hospital care and to medical specialists, where required
        Physical rehabilitation
        Mental health services
    Education or Day Programs
        Infant and preschool programs, including integration into Head Start and day
          care
        Mainstreaming in public education
        Specialty programs that vary with age and intellectual requirements

Accessible Living Environments

    At home with family
    Independent living (adult)
    Foster home
    Congregate living arrangements
        1. Shared apartments
        2. Community residences
        3. ICFs and specialized treatment units

Recreation and Socialization Activities

    After school and weekends
    Vary with age level
    Vary with level of disability

Transportation

    Training for existing system (accessible)
    Special system, e.g., minibuses for those with special needs

Table 3.1   cont.

<u>Vocational and Day Activities</u>

>Prevocational training
>Job training
>Specialized procedures for more severely retarded
>Specialized employment services for selective placement in individually
>   appropriate jobs

<u>Advocacy</u>

>Individual
>Group
>Legal
>Informal, e.g., "citizen advocacy"
>Instrumental, e.g., assistance in finding and using entitlements and appropriate
>   services

<u>Religious Activities (if desired)</u>

<u>Case Management</u>

>Family support, resource management
>Help to negotiate or gain access to "the system"
>Coordination of components into an individually appropriate plan or program

Source: Adapted from H.J. Cohen, "Trends in service delivery and treatment of the mentally retarded." *Pediatric Annals* 11, no.5 (May 1982).

4

The Quality of Life

Community service providers often consider both the mentally retarded persons and their families as the "consumers." This model of relationship is derived from the concepts of economics, a way of understanding the process of production and the marketing of commodities. There are some limits to the use of this model, however, since the marketplace is not, and cannot be, entirely free. Indeed, the aim of community services is to compensate in part for the inequality of the disabled person as a competitive consumer and to assure that he shares as a citizen in the quality of life owed to everyone, regardless of cognitive and adaptive capacity. Diversity and pluralism are inherent in our American tradition of individualism. We do not all want or like the same things, yet we all agree on the basic supports and protections necessary for maintaining life and producing a sense of belonging and a feeling of well-being. The handicapped no less than others should share in this common base.

The attitudes and values of society in general are extremely important in extending these universal requirements for human development to all members of society. Mentally retarded people, like others, can and do change as they age. The eternal child is an obsolete metaphor. This assumption means that growth is expected and that needs change with age; in an orderly sequence of development, retarded persons require different resources and interventions. Furthermore, the timing of efforts to teach certain skills or to create opportunities for self-initiated behavior can be crucial for movement toward independence. Each retarded person's different self, even though retarded, must be respected by others. This can be done through the recognition that choices and preferences are not only essential to growth and good mental health, but to the autonomy and selfhood of the individual.

A young man who took up residence in a community group home expressed his new-found pleasure of selfhood: "When I came back from work I was riding my bike home late—these two ladies, one of them says, 'Good evening sir.' I said, 'Good evening ma'am.' It made me feel good and she said, 'Nice night.' I said, 'Yes it is.'" Residential services that encourage individual growth are an essential component of a community service system for mentally retarded persons. Being independent and at home is very important for any individual's sense of identity.

The philosophy that normal patterns and conditions can be made available to retarded persons should govern the establishment of these facilities. The individual who lives there must view the residence as home, a place to be somebody. As far as possible, the house should not mark the residents or set them apart by size or architecture. A ramp or fire exit, for example, should be as inconspicuous as possible. The house should be close to the mainstream of community life and, since most of the adults cannot pass a driving test, within walking distance from some amenities. Where residents have difficulty using the community because they are confined to wheelchairs, special personnel and transportation can help them gain access to work and social activities.

Community living means being able to be different and still take part in social life. Any residential alternative should establish a normal rhythm of daily life more or less like that of the other people in the community. Normal work and leisure rhythms should approximate community patterns of work, schooling, and recreation.

The residence must be seen by the larger community as an asset. Overloading a community with facilities for the mentally retarded, particularly residential facilities, produces antagonism rather than support. The community must be aware that provision of dispersed and normal environments for people needing special services helps to make them as independent as their disabilities will allow. For current or future clients who are mentally retarded, contact with community members often provides a clearer image of what to expect.

Training self-advocates or volunteer advocates can enhance the way retarded people meet their needs in a practical and timely way, by having the advocates deal with the complex web of government entitlement programs, such as SSI, food stamps, and health services, in place of those too handicapped to be self-supporting.

In part, advocacy is directed to these new complexities. Competent adults can also assist retarded persons to increase their coping skills to secure those entitlements by themselves; to manage the responsibilities that make them competent citizens, such as paying their taxes and rent; and otherwise to stay within the law. Advocacy can enhance self-development, ordinary skills in communication, and assertiveness in taking responsibility for one's actions. This initial assistance may provide the model to enable retarded persons to become more effective advocates for themselves or, at the very least, to function more independently.

Self-Advocacy

Self-help is in the oldest American tradition. It is a value that is being passed on to many mentally retarded persons. Whenever possible, each must learn how to stand up for himself or herself. *Self-advocacy* refers to learning to speak one's own piece and, on occasion, to ask for the things one needs. This concept is especially important as a way of making sure that consumers' views are considered in establishing new services.

In the rush to deinstitutionalize large numbers of mentally retarded persons, staff sometimes ignore the clients' aspirations and choices, or fail to consider that clients have to develop skills in communicating *their* goals for living. For years physically handicapped people have articulated their demands to be in charge of their own lives. With a little help from some concerned professionals, a substantial number of retarded persons are beginning to define themselves similarly.

Conventions of mentally retarded adults have demonstrated awareness of the need to be treated as human beings—as consumers, but also as something more. "We are tired of being seen first as handicapped, or retarded, or developmentally disabled," they frequently say. "We want to be seen as *people* first." Toward this end, in some training programs in self-advocacy, mentally retarded persons train *others* to ask for the things they need.

The opportunity to receive advocacy training should be available for all retarded persons. The American Coalition of Citizens with Disabilities (ACCD) is an organization that supports the concept of self-advocacy; it has carried out several projects to advance this concept. ACCD has conducted workshops on coalition building and has provided technical assistance to handicapped individuals and groups; it has also trained disabled adults to become effective volunteer consultants on vocational and career education. Dealing primarily with physically handicapped people, ACCD has sponsored advocacy education, introducing the concept in grades 9 to 12. The purpose of this project is to teach students to be competent to gain access to the various systems they will need to use as adults to secure employment, housing, recreation, transportation, and social services.

Mentally retarded individuals also need to be educated about their rights and responsibilities as citizens. At the same time, nonhandicapped individuals need to be educated about the rights of mentally retarded and developmentally disabled persons. Advocacy training, and its complement, can have significant effects on normalizing the lives of all persons, handicapped and others.

Kevin Tracy spent half of his life in state and private institutions for the mentally retarded. Subsequently, he was employed by the Texas Association for Retarded Citizens as coordinator for their self-advocacy project. This project involved providing mentally retarded persons with a basic course of instruction about their rights as citizens and as consumers of services. Tracy has recommended that federal assistance be provided to encourage local school districts to teach those basic skills necessary for young retarded persons to use their rights fully, since the training can begin early in life.

The mentally retarded have ideas as to how programs and services, which directly serve them, should be organized. They want better community-based services to help meet their needs. "As a self-advocate," Tracy writes, "it seems to me that the main effort to form community services must be centered around developing residential services."

Many professionals who deliver community-based services would agree with Tracy. Further, many would agree that the consumer is the best person to identify what is needed and determine whether or not a program meets the client's expectations. It is surely unwise to plan programs without the direct input of clients. The issue then for consideration is not whether retarded persons should be involved, but how they can be more effectively involved in planning.

Not all mentally retarded persons are capable of playing the role of the consumer or self-advocate. The problems in communicating with profoundly or severely retarded persons clearly limit their capacity to be involved in decision-making. Furthermore, no matter how much professionals believe in the value of having clients live in the least restrictive environment, in planning they must take into account other concerns such as minimizing physical risks or social and psychological exploitation by others in the community.

One aim in community residential care is to make sure that clients get the things they need to promote their development. A person living in an intermediate care facility, for example, is entitled to active treatment, yet lower-functioning retarded people cannot always ask for what they need. These residents could be polled to find out how they feel about their living conditions. In the past, parents or other family members might have assumed an advocacy responsibility; other advocates or personal representatives might have to be assigned to guarantee that habilitation is attempted.

Advocacy

In addition to family members and court-appointed guardians, volunteers or paid case managers can function as advocates for mentally retarded persons, assisting in many needed tasks so the handicapped persons may live independently in the community. Examples include providing information on how to use a telephone, shop, or acquire food stamps. Community services systems, whether specialized or generic, are complex even for fully independent people. The situation is made more complicated when a person has limited intellectual skills and perhaps cannot even express his interests or preferences. An advocate is then faced with the problem of interpreting for him.

There are several ways of determining the interests and preferences of retarded persons who cannot advocate for themselves, and all are somewhat flawed. An advocate may consider acting in the person's "best interest," from the point of view of the advocate himself or of the family or the agency with responsibility for this particular person. This is not equivalent to independent advocacy. In this form there is no effort to make the sponsor (family, agency, or advocate) accountable for maintaining movement toward greater independence. In the "in the shoes of" approach the advocate attempts to reconstruct how a person with the characteristics of this particular retarded person would want to act *if* he could communicate his or her decision. The advocate may choose to be guided by an ideology of integration or "normalization." Herein may be found a clash of equally valid principles, as when specialized services are evidently needed and these services are not found in unrestricted or ordinary environments in schools or workplaces, or when the individual's aspirations fall short of those the advocate has for him. In taking the role of the client, the advocate may find it hard to separate his own personal preferences from how he perceives the client wants to be treated, so the personal values of the advocate may be projected onto the client. Preferences also mean giving up other valid choices. For example, the work-oriented advocate might not apply for economic assistance (to which a disabled person is legally entitled) in order to discourage the growth of dependence on the welfare system. Clearly, any approach to advocacy has its risks and should be monitored to evaluate its advantages and disadvantages.

Some mental retardation service providers in the community see themselves as primarily oriented to working with families, the predominant situation with retarded children. Case managers who assist families also may offer them training in how to negotiate the bureaucratic system and thus help themselves and their handicapped child. Training is not limited to transmitting skills that can be used for a lifetime of dealing individually with bureaucracies, because bureaucracies can be changed. Self-advocacy for families of the mentally retarded may be collective, extending to the formation of lobbies to gain services. For example, a case manager/advocate may bring parents together to lobby for after-school recreation programs for their retarded children.

Existing community services must find a way of making mentally retarded people and their families feel at home with the delivery system. Advocacy as a concept encourages that sense of partnership. The Foster Grandparents Program sponsored by ACTION, for example, matches children with special needs to older, mostly low-income adults who are prepared to commit themselves to the welfare of this population.

It is surely unscientific to generalize from the articulate statements of self-advocates like Kevin Tracy to all persons receiving mental retardation services in the community. There is certainly good reason, however, to support the sentiments expressed by his concern at the 1980 conference on community care that:

> We must look at the consumer who is regarded as a human being first and accord this human being the dignity he justly deserves. We must redirect programs and services in order that they will not continue to devalue those persons who receive these services. Rather, that services be provided, not only to meet the needs of these people who are retarded, but which also enhance the position of these persons with the full measure of dignity to which *they* as individuals are entitled [sic].

5

The Application of Decisive Technology: New Forms of Diagnosis, Treatment and Prevention

Scientific discoveries in physics and other basic sciences continually make it possible for medicine to make substantial advances. The diagnosis, treatment, and prevention of mental retardation, as a specialty within medicine, is involved in what may be called the second great scientific revolution in medicine.

The scientific foundation of modern medicine was set during the seventeenth and eighteenth centuries in rules for careful observation and by the inventions that extended the senses, such as the microscope, which made possible later discoveries of microorganisms as causes of disease. If this process were repeated in our time, we would have to redefine mental retardation, possibly eliminating the permanency of some, if not most, of the disorders under this general label.

Until the last decade, diagnosis, treatment, and prevention of mental retardation was little more than "caring for" or standing by, "a nontechnology" according to Lewis Thomas, president of Sloan Kettering Cancer Center in New York City. Less frequently found in the mental retardation field is a second order of technology that Thomas regards as costly and ineffective. Defined as "halfway technologies," these are interventions that attempt to compensate for the incapacitating effects of certain diseases about whose course little can be done. It is clear that, without fully understanding the mechanisms causing the various types of mental retardation, we cannot prevent or reverse a failure to develop cognitively and socially. Finally, the field is at the point of delivering some "decisive technologies"—relatively simple, inexpensive, and workable technologies based on the understanding of etiologies. These technologies are exemplified by modern methods of immunization and the use of antibiotics to treat bacterial infections, which, prior to effective prevention or treatment, caused sequellae including mental retardation.

The current era of advancing technology and scientific progress is having, and no doubt will continue to have, an explosive impact on service delivery for the mentally retarded. This review of new technology is not intended to be a comprehensive analysis of all technological progress in the mental retardation field, but is an attempt to identify some important developments, as well as to examine some of the problems associated with the application of new techniques. In doing so, we will focus on new discoveries and uses of current knowledge that may become the common practices in the future.

Improvements in diagnosis, prevention, and treatment of mental retardation have brought significant benefits. But the applications of technological advances have created new concerns about intervention. At issue are ethical dilemmas concerning (a) when and to whom the techniques should be applied, (b) how vigorous the life-saving or life-prolonging measures used should be, and (c) how potentially depersonalizing and dehumanizing the use of new technology may become.

A common image or perception of technological development is of economical and glamorous applications of the microprocessor to enable handicapped people to use robots for motor activities they are otherwise unable to complete. Artificial limbs and other electronically activated prosthetic devices are other obvious applications. Yet probably the greatest current and future impact of technology appears to be in advances in genetic engineering and cell biology, permitting optimistic speculation about more efficacious and astonishing prevention measures and even some dramatic cures.

Prevention and Treatment

Prevention is an area in which the use of new techniques has burgeoned in the past decade and which holds considerable promise for the future.

ANTENATAL

In the 1950s and early 1960s, two important occurrences revolutionized the field of antenatal diagnosis. The first was the ability to detect chromosomal abnormalities, both in terms of number and, subsequently, gross structure and composition. The second was amniocentesis, first applied to detect and treat cases of hyperbilirubinemia due to RH blood incompatibility and then, subsequently, to identify chromosomal abnormalities and a variety of metabolic disorders. These developments led to the current, almost routinely accepted screening of the fetuses of at-risk pregnant mothers for disorders such as Down's Syndrome (in which an extra chromosome or extra part of a chromosome is present), and to make the antenatal diagnosis of types of neural tube defects by detecting abnormally high levels of alpha fetoprotein in the amniotic fluid. The capability also exists to identify many types of chromosomal or hereditary metabolic disorders. More recently, chorionic biopsies are being utilized or tested as an antenatal diagnostic methodology that may be more effective than amniocentesis, and refined imaging techniques such as ultrasound (the most widely used noninvasive apparently benign procedure) are being used to identify abnormal physical characteristics of the developing fetus. Computerized X-rays or Nuclear Magnetic Resonance are other important diagnostic techniques. These procedures are now being supplemented by methods of directly visualizing fetal structures (fetoscopy) using fiber optic instruments that are introduced via amniocentesis, and by obtaining direct blood samples from infants while visualized using the above described methodology.

The improvements in our capability in antenatal diagnosis have led not only to the option of termination of pregnancy in cases of abnormalities of the fetus, a solution frought with obvious serious ethical dilemmas, but also to some advances in treatment. In the latter area scientists have barely scratched the surface. In recent years, fetal surgery has been performed to treat hydrocephalous, a condition in which increased pressure and amount of fluid in the ventricles of the brain, if untreated, may progressively compromise brain functioning. Other vital organ systems that may be progressively damaged in utero are also accessible to surgical intervention. The adverse effects of blood incompatibilities have also been successfully treated in utero. The potential exists and is already being utilized for in utero treatment of some metabolic disorders, and also for their immediate treatment after birth. Such treatment aims at maximum preservation of brain and other organ functioning in the fetuses and infants.

PERINATAL

Rapid strides have been made in the identification of metabolic disorders at birth since the initial introduction of ferric chloride testing of diapers in the mid-1950s, followed by the use of the innovative mass-screening techniques for Phenylketonuria (PKU) by Guthrie in 1961. Widespread application followed of automated mandatory metabolic screening programs for neonates, organized by state or region, for the identification of up to seven metabolic disorders, including PKU, hypothyroidism, galactosemia, homocystinuria, tyrosinemia, maple syrup urine disease, and histidinemia. While screening for hypothyroidism and PKU have relatively high yields of 1 to 3000–4,000 and 1 to 10,000–15,000 respectively, the other metabolic disorders are rarer. In addition, the greatest successes thus far have been noted in the treatment of the two most common conditions: very early introduction of special diets are helping PKU children, and thyroid medications are effectively improving the prognosis for infants with congenital hypothyroidism. Despite the relatively low yield of cases from screening, the treatment successes and long-term cost savings, plus the relatively low cost of such screening procedures, have encouraged the widespread application of infant metabolic screening programs. As new techniques are developed and perfected to identify pathological conditions, screening programs will be expanded, particularly for diseases with more common occurrences.

INSTRUMENTATION AND MONITORING

Another important area of prevention in the perinatal period, aided by technological development, is the improvement of instrumentation and monitoring, as applied to high-risk situations, both during labor and after birth. Thus far, monitoring of high risk pregnancies during labor has proved to be a somewhat mixed blessing, since it may generate unnecessary treatments. The monitoring records infant heart rate and changes in intrauterine pressure during labor to detect signs of fetal distress. While this widely applied procedure clearly identifies some infants who require rapid, immediate delivery to avoid possible death or sequellae such as brain damage, one unintended consequence is a rapid rise in Cesarean Section rates at some hospitals. Any deviation from normal detected by the monitoring may be incorrectly interpreted by anxious obstetricians who, fearful of potential litigous parents who would blame them for an abnormal offspring, may more quickly exercise the option of a surgical delivery and thus contribute to abnormally high rates of Cesarean Sections. National experts have indicated a need for improved prenatal monitoring techniques, more research on the implications of deviations from normal patterns, and better training of personnel who utilize monitoring devices. These recommendations lead to the conclusion that further improvements in monitoring techniques and more effective use of the information obtained are likely occurrences in the future.

The other area of considerable interest at present is the monitoring of prematures and newborns from both physiological and behavioral standpoints. One has only to visit a hospital unit caring for premature babies or a Neonatal Intensive Care Unit (NICU) to recognize the revolution that technology has wrought. Cluttered with oscilloscopes, beepers, equipment for ventilatory assistance, and other electronic hardware, the NICUs resemble something out of the space program. Incubators are equipped with instruments to measure oxygen and temperature levels. The infant's pulse, respiratory, and arterial oxygen levels are measured by sensing devices, the latest being skin-attached and of a noninvasive nature. All of these devices are honed to (a) assure the baby of an optimum oxygen supply to permit normal brain development (but not too much to cause retrolental fibroplasia, a potentially disabling eye condition that once was a common problem among premature infants receiving too much oxygen); (b) achieve optimum temperature and humidity levels to minimize insensitive water loss while stabilizing the infant's metabolic status; and (c) detect signs of danger or illness signaled by changes in the infant's heart or respiratory rates. Infants are maintained in biological balance through the use of blood tests that require small drops of blood samples for automated microanalytic clinical analyses, and biochemical inbalances are corrected through the use of electronically regulated and monitored infusions of intravenous fluids.

ASSISTED VENTILATION

A dramatic mode of intervention that has grown in use during the past decade, mechanical devices can assist infants with their breathing and oxygen exchange. Assisted ventilation is accepted practice in premature units and NICUs and has saved many lives and prevented serious neurological sequellae in others. An aura of ethical controversy surrounds its use, however, centering on the management of very low birth weight infants with associated problems, who may, with the help of advanced and costly technology, survive a stormy and lengthy hospital stay only to later become multiply handicapped children who are a burden to their families and to society. Still unresolved is the fundamental issue of how to decide and who should be involved in determining how heroic such interventions should be.

Similar difficult questions are found in the controversy around the provision of extensive life support measures for the deformed full-term or premature baby, the very tiny premature infant with a poor prognosis, or the child with severe acquired brain damage due to trauma or illness. Technology has enabled physicians to maintain respiration and heart beats in infants and children with a terrible prognosis for normal brain functioning. But for how long should this be provided? Since resources are limited, for whom should they be provided? Who will make these decision? What is government's role? What is the family's role? Are economic consideration important? There are no simple answers to these questions.

We hope that research will provide techniques to improve our ability to predict future problems or, better still, to prevent them from occurring in the first place. In the meantime, the advancements in technology have presented us with new perplexing quandaries for which acceptable management strategies have yet to be developed.

EARLY IDENTIFICATION OF DISABILITIES

Early diagnosis of developmental abnormalities has recently been extended through innovative methods that measure physiological processes. Appearing in the past decade, the most notable of these advances involve the testing of auditory and visual functioning through evoked responses. These techniques, which respectively test brain stem and cortical functioning, provide a stimulus to a suspect infant being screened for a sensory disorder and use computer averaging of the electroencephalographic (EEG) responses to detect deviations from normal. While the use of EEGs as a diagnostic instrument is not new, the refinement of evoked response testing aided by sophisticated computer programs is a more recent event. In addition, computerized averaging of infant heart and respiratory rates, as well as determinations of changes in amplitude and quality, are all being used by researchers to detect disturbances in autonomic functioning of the nervous system or other areas of neurological dysfunction.

While the application of automation and computers to physiological research has proceeded rapidly, their use in behavioral analysis is more problematic. Human observers are still required to test and evaluate the responses of newborns and young children. Yet computer-assisted analysis of the data produced is a valuable aid to behavioral researchers. The latter investigators have, as a result, produced and refined screening instruments such as the Brazelton Neonatal Behavioral Scales or the Einstein Neonatal Behavioral Assessment Scale, which are useful in detecting some abnormalities in young infants. Nonetheless, the predictability of these instruments in forecasting later developmental problems remains uncertain. Despite these defects, it should be noted that investigators are striving to perfect screening and assessment instruments using computerized analysis of data to determine at a later age which components of the tests are most effective and/or reliable.

Imaging Devices

Dramatic changes in the capability to diagnose both structural and physiological abnormalities of the brain have come about through the development of new and very elegant computerized imaging devices. The first, best known, and most widely applied is Computerized Tomography, or what is commonly known as CT or CAT scans. This methodology involves taking X-rays from all angles to create a cross-sectional image of the brain. Permitting a three-dimensional view of the brain, the procedure enables the examiner to detect developmental abnormalities in brain structure, tumors, abnormalities in the size of the ventricles (the fluid containing compartments in the brain), or hemorrhages. The latter is particularly useful in diagnosing the sequellae of trauma, and ventricular size is important in monitoring the development or treatment of hydrocephalous.

Another important device that creates similar images of brain structure and does not require use of radiation is ultrasound tomography. Rapidly growing and widely used, ultrasound imaging, based on measurement of acoustic impedance, detects not only the physical features of the in utero fetus, but also can examine high-risk neonates for signs of brain hemorrhage, a common complication among very low birth weight infants or others with severe respiratory problems.

Two other exciting instruments that are just beginning to be used in clinical settings are Nuclear Magnetic Resonance (NMR) and Positron Emission Tomography (PET) scanners. The first, an excellent technique for visualizing soft tissue structures including the brain, depends on the use of a strong magnetic field to change the alignment of oscillating hydrogen atoms in water and other materials of the body so that protons line up with the magnetic field and an image is produced reflecting the density and composition of the structure. The net result is a set of images like CT scanning but without using radiation. PET scanning is based on detection of gamma radiation from isotopes. It can be used to detect cellular and intracellular functioning when any positron-emitting isotopes of carbon, nitrogen, oxygen, and fluorine are involved. It detects concentrations of different radionucletides and can produce magnificent multicolor images to illustrate metabolic functions, including the flow of substances or sites of receptor concentration. It offers very profound research possibilities in determining the biochemical changes that occur under normal circumstances and in abnormal conditions. These techniques are so new that their clinical applications remain to be defined. But their use offers marvelous opportunities to enhance our knowledge about the physiology, pathology, and possible treatment modalities for brain dysfunctions, including mental retardation.

Uses of Automation for the Physically Handicapped

The development and refinement of the microprocessor and improved understanding of physiology have led to the burgeoning of the field of innovative prosthetic devices. Communication devices using computer technology and scanners for nonverbal or augmentative communication are probably the most widely used inventions. Artificial conveyances such as wheelchairs, with special capabilities including electric power, are commonplace, and advanced models will soon be able to climb stairs. The large battery packs make such wheelchairs heavy, another problem still to be solved. Artificial limbs, improved by use of modern plastics and equipped with electronic gadgetry, make prostheses more efficient. Devices that will actually "walk" the paraplegic individual are currently being demonstrated. Also in experimental stages are sensory devices that can be implanted in blind people to interpret visual inputs and transmit these to the brain to simulate seeing. Research is proceeding on similar auditory sensing devices at the same time that microelectronics has reduced the size and possible cosmetic shortcomings of hearing aids, while improving the sound quality transmitted.

Another area in which the microprocessor promises to aid the mentally retarded is the use of microcomputers as instructional devices. When used as a teaching aid, a contingency intervention system is applied in which correct responses are reinforced by positive feedback from the microcomputer. This type of approach has reportedly proved successful with learning disabled and some mildly retarded individuals, but its application to the more severely retarded is more limited. One recalls the hopes raised by the introduction of the talking typewriter to reinforce autistic children so they could make academic gains, an approach which did little to improve their social interaction, a very serious deficit in autistic children. The same concern may apply to mentally retarded children and adults where any learning format that does not promote social skills development has serious drawbacks.

On the horizon is the potential use of robots to assist retarded and/or physically handicapped individuals to perform functions that are otherwise beyond their capability. It has been projected that the use of automation will reduce the staff time required for direct care functions and make both community and institutional care less costly. These benefits have yet to be demonstrated. Listening devices and TV cameras are widely used in hospitals to monitor client functioning, and were introduced in the 1970s to other types of facilities. The advantage of listening or looking out for client problems from a central location is particularly beneficial in the presence of staff shortages. Nevertheless, these devices have been criticized on the grounds that they constitute an invasion of privacy, decrease one-to-one contact with staff, and depersonalize care. The latter criticism also applies to the use of robots as client aids, when the major needs of the handicapped individuals are to learn new skills themselves and become more independent, rather than becoming more dependent; to improve social skills; and to learn appropriate behavior from real life role models.

Telecommunication

The explosion in communications technology has fostered potential applications in the biomedical sciences and in social services. Telemetric monitoring of brain and cardiac functioning is a routine procedure in some medical centers. Electronic mail systems now speed communications between users and can disseminate new information almost instantaneously. One of the earliest uses of this means of rapid communication in the mental retardation and developmental disability field was the system installed by the national network of University Affiliated Facilities and Programs (UAFs). These university-based programs organized an electronic mail system in the late 1970s to foster collaborative information-gathering activities, joint program development efforts, and dissemination of new findings. The network primarily focused on expanding training and research activities. In recent years, state Developmental Disability Councils, federal offices, and state Maternal and Child Health agencies were added to the network.

Concomitant with the establishment of the electronic mail system, UAFs conducted other telecommunication experiments. Among these was a program in Vermont that provided a telephone linkage between families of disabled children and to the UAF affiliated service agency, permitting teleconferencing among groups of parents and assistance when needed from a service provider. The experiment proved to be very successful. A second experiment used television hookups at four locations scattered throughout the United States to offer regional workshops, with visual materials transmitted to distant cites from a central location.

The use of new communications technology is clearly in its infancy. Computers linked by modems to central data sources will, in the future, be commonplace in homes of professionals and consumers, and have potential as educational tools for staff and/or clients. Interactive cable systems may permit program demonstrations or lectures followed by question-and-answer sessions for consumers or professionals. Group telephone conferencing between professionals and parents will result in significant savings of travel costs and time expended by all participants.

Yet the application of this technology, as well as other scientific advances, is not without potential problems. Despite its potential advantage of reaching people at distant locations, substitution of a screen or a telephone for direct contact can lead to depersonalization in the provision of human services. Furthermore, not everyone is trained to use or feels comfortable with computers and telephone conferencing modes of communication, although this shortcoming will be reduced in the coming years as the younger generation, bred in the newer technologies, becomes the primary user and the current high cost of equipment lessens. Nevertheless, the dangers remain that rapid advances in communications technology can enhance the gap between people with normal capabilities and those individuals with limited cognitive abilities who cannot master the newer, complex systems that will be developed in the future.

Studying the Future

In addition to the areas of technology already described, some new ones are being mentioned in preliminary reports in scientific journals. One area pertinent to the prevention of mental retardation is the role of toxic agents in the environment. Current research has already extended the knowledge base far beyond the known harmful substances, such as the heavy metals and insecticides. Posing interesting research questions are the impact of many other substances on in utero development and subsequent behavior, and advances in our capability to detect potential pollutants, additives, and other noxious substances in the environment, coupled with research on their effects. The use of biological markers to verify an exposure to toxic substances is still a new, relatively unexplored area. These studies will no doubt be aided by techniques such as PET scanning and should permit greater understanding of what substances promote or inhibit brain functioning.

Another area of future research that relates to improvement in brain functioning is development of memory-enhancing medications or even specialized dietary changes. Investigations relating to Alzheimer's Disease, a late complication of Down's Syndrome and a major problem for the general aging population in the United States, should help determine the physiology and chemistry of memory and how to restore and improve it. This drug research should have beneficial spinoffs to those working with the mentally retarded.

While we can envision significant advances as a result of NMR and PET scanning devices, the use of other computer aided diagnostic techniques is also likely. Attempts at mapping areas of brain function will no doubt be aided by devices such as the Brain State Analyzer or BEAM (brain electrical activity mapping), which evaluates the quality and quantity of brain electrical activity under a variety of circumstances and produces colorful printouts or maps of areas of brain function, while apparently illustrating the localization of neurological dysfunction.

Finally, no discussion of the use of new technology would be complete without mention of organ transplants and genetic engineering. According to a recent review article in *Science*, neurologists have been studying transplantation techniques for many years in amphibians, fish, and birds to learn more about brain development. Actual tissue grafts have been performed in these species and are practical tools for tackling unsolved problems of mammalian behavior and brain development. Successful transplantation of fetal brain tissue has been a particular area of interest in studying brain and neuronal development. The success of animal work has already led to attempts by Swedish scientists to treat humans with Parkinson's disease, a disease of the basal ganglia, by injections of tissue capable of producing the required substances to remedy the underlying chemical deficiency and thereby improve functioning. While this type of approach has been successful in animals, the results in humans are still uncertain. One interesting observation thus far is that brain graft rejections are unlikely to occur. Whether this results in functional improvement will be the critical issue. Nonetheless, the use of brain tissue transplants is clearly in its infancy, and its potential for dealing with deficits in brain functioning is impossible to predict. A considerable number of technical problems makes its extensive use unlikely in the foreseeable future.

An area in which activity is widespread, but clinical applications are still few, is genetic engineering. The ability to transfer genes from one species to the next is a remarkable achievement of the past decade, and the potential applications to biology, botany, and bacteriology are legion. The few clinical applications already achieved are in the use of bacteria, modified by engineered insertion of genetic material, to produce large quantities of substances such as insulin, interferon, or growth hormone. These substances would otherwise have to be extracted from human or animal tissues. The potential applications to the field of mental retardation primarily revolve around the possible treatment of inborn errors of metabolism such as PKU or Lipoidoses, the former an example of a disorder currently requiring major expense and changes in lifestyle to treat, and the latter being one group among many examples of currently untreatable progressive conditions. Insertion of a gene to correct the causative metabolic defect, usually a missing enzyme, would totally change the approach to treatment or management of these disorders. The insertion of a gene into cells to correct the metabolic disorder Lesch-Nyhan Syndrome, a disorder with severe mental retardation and self-destructive behavior, has been achieved in vitro. But it is a long way from the in vitro manufacture of a substance in bacteria or even humans to producing changes in the cellular functioning of human beings in vivo. Yet such changes are possible and likely in the future, if experiments with genetic engineering, despite the weighty ethical questions involved, are permitted to continue.

Conclusion

Technological advances have already brought about many changes in the diagnosis and treatment of the mentally retarded. The area of prevention has clearly benefited, and new efforts in genetic engineering expand everyone's hopes for the future. It is not beyond the realm of possibility that not only genetic, but total chromosomal engineering, as would be required to prevent Down's Syndrome, could be accomplished. Advances in imaging techniques, EEG technology, and microanalytic chemistry as applied to metabolic screening have all contributed to improved capability for making earlier and more accurate diagnoses that lead to the earlier and more effective treatment. Treatment approaches are likely to be assisted by the use of sophisticated automated equipment, which also bring concomitant ethical dilemmas. Technology is sometimes seen as a substitute for social learning. Robots may be potential labor-saving devices or they may provide improved mobility when there is a motor problem. But except when used in situations where they aid communication or make interpersonal contact more likely, robots are unlikely to promote social growth among individuals who sorely need enhanced social competence.

While technology and science continue to march on, it is evident that those applying the advanced technology have not made comparable progress in confronting or resolving the moral and ethical problems that the changes have brought.

Part Two

Service Planning, Administration, and Funding

6

The Politics of Mental Retardation: History, Legislation and Policy Making

Introduction

The costs of health care, particularly for individuals with chronic physical or mental illness and for the mentally retarded, are now undergoing close scrutiny. Concerns about the inflationary impact of massive federal budget deficits, rapid growth of federal entitlement programs, and other financial uncertainties have increased competition for limited resources.

Fiscal concerns clearly have political implications. Still, other significant factors have contributed to the apparent politicization of the health and mental health fields. Among these are the growth of the consumer movement and an increasingly vocal constituency; the interest of numerous professional groups and organizations; the concerns for jobs on the part of unions; the interest of the human rights advocates; the passage of important new legislation; the courts' interpretation of the laws or the Constitution, and the resolution of local disputes that determine who is entitled to what; and, finally, the mass media's tendency to use sensationalism as a means of commanding audience attention, thereby focusing on the exposure of the abuses and evils of large residential institutions in the service system.

The interplay of these factors has raised the level of expectations on the part of consumers (mostly parents), legislators, and elements of the public that positive changes could be achieved. But when immediate improvements were not forthcoming, it also increased the level of tension among competing elements or groups. When failures occur, scapegoats are sought to explain why change has not been accomplished, efficient use of resources not achieved, and the seemingly inevitable scandals associated with large congregate care institutional facilities not eliminated. Consequently, there is a high turnover in leadership positions, particularly among those overseeing or administering state institutional systems and their individual facilities.

To understand the political tensions that now exist, it is useful to examine the evolution of the community's and the government's commitment to managing the problems of the mentally retarded. The commitment to provide services of any kind historically followed both the development of interventions for other handicapped persons and the politically popular views existing at that time. In other words, differing handicaps have been responded to in a different manner and in a different order as exemplified by the discussion of the federal entitlement programs later in this chapter. This pattern confirms the view that society at various times has regarded some types of disabled individuals and their families as more deserving of assistance than others.

Along with the growing appreciation of the fact that handicapped persons can benefit from rehabilitation, there have been cycles of support for the idea that those who are disabled because of some mental, rather than physical, condition are capable of living normal lives in the community. Beliefs about the mentally retarded shifted markedly around the turn of the century. The widespread mid-nineteenth century view that training the mentally retarded in separate facilities could restore intelligence changed to the late nineteenth and early twentieth century belief that they were beyond any form of rehabilitation and, therefore, a menace to society.

An Historical Survey

Prior to the middle of the nineteenth century, the mentally retarded, both in Europe and the United States, were accorded special treatment in public facilities only if they were also indigent. In general, specialized residential schools were created for them following similar efforts for the blind, deaf, and insane. The facilities tended to accumulate unwanted children or adults, usually indigent, or social outcasts, who were either illiterate, had odd behavior, were epileptic, or had physical handicaps. In the early literature on facilities not much is said about caring for what would now be considered the severely and profoundly mentally retarded. The development of the public residential care facility for the mentally retarded and other deviant populations is a phenomenon of the Western world. It appears to reflect the evolution of the concept of a public responsibility for the deviant, afflicted, or the subnormal.

The first publicly supported U.S. asylum for the mentally retarded was established in Massachusetts in 1850, with New York State opening a similar facility a year later. These efforts were not a result of broad support for provision of institutional care in these industrialized states. In 1845, a report had been made to the New York State legislature that estimated the number of cases in the state and discussed methods employed in treating mentally retarded persons in Europe. Subsequently, a bill was offered for the creation of an institution, but it passed only one part of the bicameral government.

Six years later, the legislature approved an "experimental school," subsequently housed in a rented building in Albany. Permanency was achieved in 1853 when donated land in Syracuse became the home of the first state school in New York.

Sources of support for state training schools, as they became known, were selective, coming mainly from physicians, teachers, clergy, and women's clubs. Supporters of these early programs believed training would make the retardate a normal person. To justify this belief, administrators of state training schools tended to select high-level mentally retarded persons to demonstrate that their care was effective. The first age group selected for these programs were children who were trained and legally required to be released between age sixteen and twenty. When it became evident that training would not rehabilitate all of the retarded, the age of release was extended and finally left to the discretion of the superintendent. Custodial orientations were first evident in the changes in legal requirements affecting female patients, thereby avoiding their release during child-bearing years.

When first established, however, the state training schools were rehabilitative in orientation. In keeping with the wave of charitable sentiment toward the handicapped in the United States in the 1850s, a variety of professional and popular writers supported the establishment of institutions to educate the handicapped. Editorials in progressive journals and general magazines called for provisions for the disabled, including the mentally retarded.

In the following decades, the accomplishments of the state training schools for the mentally retarded were regarded as disappointing. By the 1870s, the stress on rehabilitation was being replaced by an emphasis on custodial care—a form of protection for both the defective person and society. By the end of the century, professional and popular opinion regarded the mentally retarded as a dangerous class. Specifically, the higher-level mentally retarded were defined as a source of social problems as diverse as crime and illegitimacy. Writing in the *Popular Science Monthly*, an editor in 1898 evaluated the older perspective, stating that: "The idea is foolish that training can prepare even those of higher grades to battle with the world and fit them for a life outside of institutional walls."

Colonies set apart from the rest of society were recommended by the superintendents of state schools as the best way of dealing with the problem. In monasticlike surroundings, the mentally retarded would be trained to lead useful lives.

> Here [those so qualified] separated from the world and forbidden to marry shall become self-supporting, self-respecting citizens, who are in full possession of an assured freedom—always with careful direction and supervision, and a degree of independence in lieu of degradation and ignominy. [Proceedings of Medical Officers of American Institutions for Idiots and Feebleminded Persons, 1897, p. 3.]

The medical officers were supported by the social work professionals. The 1894 National Conference of Charities and Correction said that the establishment of colonies would provide a useful way of controlling the mentally retarded:

> The benefits to society of replacing a wholly unproductive class is certainly something to be counted. The removal of an irresponsible and dangerous class from the floating population is much more to be considered as a boon to society. The advantage which must accrue from the close limiting and extensive reduction of this class is greatest of all, and sufficient to warrant a greater expenditure of public funds than has ever been demanded.

By 1915, this same conference regarded the control of the mentally retarded as a vital concern. Gone were the rehabilitation benefits of institutional care; the only concern was containment of a danger:

> For many generations we have recognized and pitied the idiot. Of late we have recognized a higher type of defective, the moron, and have discovered that he is a burden, that he is a menace to society and civilization, that he is responsible in large degree for many if not all of our social problems.

Additional support for the idea of containment came from the eugenics movement and some mental hygiene societies formed locally in the United States. In the first two decades of the twentieth century, these organizations advocated not only custodial care, but also sterilization for the mentally retarded, to prevent increasing numbers who would be a burden to the commonweal. This concern for the protection of society led to the eventual passage of sterilization laws in the large majority of states.

Despite these views, efforts were made as early as 1896 to include the mentally retarded in community school programs. Starting in Providence, Rhode Island, school classes for mildly retarded children, also known as educable retarded, were created in eleven cities during the last few years of the century. By the 1950s, the professional view was that mental retardation left its mark throughout a person's lifetime, requiring a broad continuum of services for the purposes of adequate prevention, treatment and care. But it took the development of legislative support for other disabled persons and the self-help efforts of parents of mentally retarded children to accelerate the trend toward community care.

THE IMPETUS FOR EARLY LEGISLATIVE CHANGE

Community care or services for the mentally retarded followed the development of innovations in rehabilitating the physically disabled. The first sheltered workshops were created for the blind in the 1930s; these efforts soon received federal subsidies. People with other disabilities were found to be also capable of working in sheltered settings or of being retrained for employment in the labor market.

The justification for rehabilitation and community services, instead of inactivity or long-term hospitalization, came from the consequences of World War II. Many returning veterans, whose lives were saved by battlefield surgery, refused to remain hidden from public view in chronic disease hospitals as charity cases. In addition, the greater availability of prosthetic devices for amputees, coupled with low-cost automobiles and fuel, made it possible for thousands of wheelchair-bound people, or those on crutches, to become mobile.

The post–World War II era brought about other substantial nationwide changes that accelerated the development of services for the mentally retarded. One important development was the civil rights movement, an early component of the broader human rights movement of which the rights of the handicapped and mentally retarded became a later, but significant, component. A second change was the creation of consumerism as an element in American society, in which the quality of services and products and how they affected families and their offspring became an important issue. Consumers became more activist in their willingness to lobby for improvements or changes in services. A third, more general element was the overall economic improvement and escalated demands for an improved quality of life for families, workers, and all elements of society as the United States (and other countries) emerged from the suffering of the Depression, followed by the scourge of World War II. The latter historical occurrence, particularly the horrors caused by Nazi racial theories, combined with the ideology of the civil rights movement, increased revulsion to or at least criticism of the theories of genetic inferiority. Thus, a rekindled belief in giving all people a fair chance encouraged the development of the service structure for the mentally retarded.

As a result of these influences, many families who had been limited to two service options for their retarded child or relative—placement in a large institution, or remaining at home with no services or programs except the limited availability of special education classes—now demanded, and were given, other choices.

It is of interest that changes in the care of the mentally ill also impacted on the mentally retarded. In almost all states until the late 1960s and 1970s, services for the mentally retarded and mentally ill were housed in departments of mental hygiene or another umbrella agency of a similar or a broader type. Mental hygiene agencies were almost always directed by psychiatrists, and state institutions for the mentally retarded were also usually directed by psychiatrists. This psychiatric control of programs for the mentally retarded evolved from the classification of the mentally retarded as deviant or unable to control their mental functions, characteristics usually attributed to the mentally ill. When the concept of an asylum or other segregated place was applied to the mentally ill, it was simultaneously applied to the mentally retarded, and similar types of facilities were made available to them. Both populations required considerable care over a long period of time. In fact, in the past many state hospitals housed both mentally ill and mentally retarded individuals, and some have continued to do so until the present time.

Although the psychiatric literature in the twentieth century has infrequent mention of the mentally retarded, the profession of psychiatry continued to retain responsibility for their oversight, care, and treatment. Part of this relates to the professional views that were common in the field. As Sarason pointed out in the preface to Burton Blatt's *Christmas in Purgatory*, we have employed a self-fulfilling prophecy in our conceptual approach to psycho-pathology in regarding the mentally retarded or the schizophrenic as incapable of improvement. He added:

> that most of these patients did not improve and did not reflect the validity of the diagnosis, but the dishearteningly effective way in which state hospitals unwittingly went about confirming their diagnosis.

A second reason was the accepted belief that both populations have chronic brain syndromes. Consequently, psychiatrists were considered expert in neurology and brain function; and this expertise made them the appropriate overseer of care for mentally retarded as well as the mentally ill.

The final reason was the desire of bureaucracies and those in control to maintain the status quo. No doubt many in the psychiatric establishment truly viewed themselves either as the profession of choice or, in the words of Steven Marcus in his essay on the development of the English poorhouses in *Doing Good—The Limits of Benevolence*, as being "their brother's keepers." In the same volume, Glasser points out in his essay "Prisoners of Benevolence" that well-intentioned protective mechanisms were distorted into procedures that denied clients rights by mental health or child care officials, who saw their discretion being limited or jobs threatened by proposed changes in the systems in which they worked. Self-preservation all too often appeared to become the guiding motive for bureaucrats or administrators of this system of care. Psychiatry, through control over the mental hygiene system, continued to dominate the mental retardation field, despite the rapid decline during the twentieth century in the number of psychiatrists choosing to work in state hospitals or institutions for the mentally retarded.

Some conceptual innovations in the field of psychiatry in the 1950s and 1960s did have a positive impact on services for the mentally retarded. Because of the close relationship between services for the mentally ill and the mentally retarded, when the philosophy of care for the emotionally disturbed changed to a more community-oriented approach, similar improvements were applied to the mentally retarded.

Conventional wisdom in the medical profession once held that people with psychiatric histories or those in state hospitals could not take care of themselves in the community and would continue to require institutiona-lization in isolated settings. But in the 1950s, the idea surfaced that the social environment had a substantial impact on the behavior of normal people *and* on those with psychiatric histories. A new concept in psychiatric care developed, leading to the creation of a therapeutic community. It was reasoned that if psychiatric patients were treated with respect, they would begin to take control over their own lives. In addition, the development of major tranquilizing drugs, such as thorazine, made it possible to limit some of the acute psychotic behavior of psychiatric patients, leading psychiatrists to conclude that these patients could also be managed in the community.

In the same era, professionals and parents began to believe that within a proper therapeutic milieu at home or in specialized community-based facilities, if treated more normally and offered special treatment where needed, the mentally retarded would benefit from living in the community; they would show functional improvements and behave more normally. As a result, parents of handicapped children started programs for children who had been excluded from public schools because of the belief that the disabled could not benefit from education with nonhandicapped children. The desire to live a more normal life helped mothers of disabled children to overcome any hesitations in starting organizations to provide services that were unavailable elsewhere. In so doing, they helped to create a climate of greater tolerance for all the disabled in society. In this spirit of self-help, parent-run voluntary associations were formed throughout the United States. These led to creation of state parent associations for the mentally retarded and eventually to a national organization, the National Association for Retarded Children, now called the Association for Retarded Citizens. This organization is the largest consumer association of its type in the United States. To fill service gaps, these consumer organizations began to create educational programs for retarded children. Later, since their offspring were excluded from sheltered workshops for the physically disabled and because of evident need, these same parents initiated sheltered workshop programs.

In 1953, the various state divisions of vocational rehabilitation were legally mandated under federal statute (P.L. 83-565) to subsidize the rehabilitation of mentally retarded people for the purpose of making them "fit to engage in a remunerative occupation." Typically, the creation of a separate workshop facility was required before individuals classified in this disability category could be trained, because other programs would not accept them. Even among the mentally retarded, state regulations limited eligibility according to aptitude. Later, federal legislation, through P.L. 88-333, made it possible to attempt rehabilitation of even relatively low-functioning mentally retarded adults, provided that they could be placed permanently in a sheltered workshop rather than in competitive employment. (See Table 6.1 for a review of all federal legislation pertaining to the mentally retarded in the community and institutional care).

THE KENNEDY ERA

The Kennedy administration promoted psychologic, legislative, and programmatic changes for the mentally retarded. The public anouncement that the president of the United States had a retarded sister, and that this prominent first family did not hide the fact, was a heartening development for families with a mentally retarded relative. Until that time, "closeted" retarded children and relatives were commonplace, since families often felt shame and guilt and were fearful of being stigmatized, perhaps from a genetic perspective, by an intolerant or unsympathetic society. The legislative and programmatic changes were the direct result of presidential

Table 6.1 Key Mental Retardation and Development Disability—Related Legislation

Year	Public law number	Title or name of legislation	Principal components
1935	P.L. 74–271	Social Security Act	Established National Social Security with income security and financial relief for needy citizens, including children. Established Maternal and Child Health and Crippled Children's Program.
1953	P.L. 83–565	Vocational Rehabilitation Act	Mandated state vocational rehabilitation to subsidize vocational rehab. agencies for the mentally retarded.
1954	P.L. 83–531	The Cooperative Research in Education Act	Authorized support for Educational Research, including for the mentally retarded
1958	P.L. 85–926	Higher Education Training Act	Provided support to private and nonprofit institutions of higher learning for training teachers, including traineeships to work with the retarded.
1963	P.L. 88–156	Maternal and Child Health and Mental Retardation Planning Amendments to the Social Security Act.	Amended Maternal and Child Health Provisions to include comprehensive maternity and infant care aimed at high-risk mothers, and authorized funds for state planning of M.R. services, including prevention activities.
1963	P.L. 88–164	Mental Retardation Facilities and Community Mental Health Center Construction Act	First major program to construct facilities for the mentally ill and retarded. Provided 75% of the cost of building Mental Retardation Research Centers and University Affiliated Facilities; grants to construct state and local facilities for the mentally retarded and Community Mental Health Centers for the mentally ill.
1964	P.L. 88–333	Rehabilitation Act Amendments	Extended eligibility for vocational rehabilitation to low-functioning mentally retarded adults.

Table 6.1 cont.

Year	Public law number	Title or name of legislation	Principal components
1965	P.L. 89–10	Elementary and Secondary Education Act	Title I assistance to educate disadvantaged children.
1965	P.L. 89–97	Amendments to the Social Security Act	Began Medicare for elderly (Title XVIII) and incorporated Medicaid (Title XIX) into the Social Security Act.
1965	P.L. 89–313	Education Amendments	Authorized assistance to handicapped children in state-operated or -supported day and residential schools.
1969	P.L. 91–230	Education of the Handicapped Act	Assisted expansion of educational programs for the handicapped.
1970	P.L. 91–517	Developmental Disabilities Services and Facilities Construction Act	Added the term "Developmental Disabilities" (D.D.) to the original Mental Retardation Act and defined D.D.; continued University Affiliated Facilities; stressed interdisciplinary training; established a formula grant program for the states with a State Planning Council with 1/3 consumers having oversight over the program; established a National Advisory Council and authorized funding for projects of National Significance.
1971	P.L. 92–233	Amendments to the Social Security Act	Authorized reimbursement for Medicaid-eligible clients in public institutions for the mentally retarded (ICF-MR program)
1972	P.L. 92–603	Amendments to the Social Security Act	Amended Title XVI to provide supplemental security payments (SSI) for the deaf, blind, and disabled.

Year	P.L.	Title	Description
1973	P.L. 93–112	Rehabilitation Act of 1973	Section 504 Regulations issued in 1977 prohibited discrimination by making it illegal to exclude disabled people from any program receiving federal funds.
1974	P.L. 93–380	Education Amendments	Required States to plan for education services for all handicapped children.
1975	P.L. 93–647	Social Security Amendment	Established Title XX program replacing Titles IVA and VI of the Social Security Act; broadened eligibility for social services and gave states greater flexibility in their administration and coordination.
1975	P.L. 94–103	Developmentally Disabled Assistance and Bill of Rights Act	Continued support for UAFs; included new Bill of Rights provision to safeguard and protect rights of D.D. persons. Added autism and conditions closely related to mental retardation to a modified definition. Required a study of the definition leading to suggestions for further change, if needed; created Protection and Advocacy systems.
1975	P.L. 94–142	The Education for All Handicapped Children's Act	Mandated free public education for all handicapped children in the least restrictive environment.
1978	P.L. 95–602	Rehabilitation, Comprehensive Services, and Developmental Disabilities Amendments of 1978	Adapted a functional definition of developmental disabilities; merged D.D. into the Rehabilitation Act and retained its other components along with vocational rehabilitation programs; encouraged comprehensive agencies for independent living; created the National Institute for Handicapped Research.

initiatives. A panel of mental retardation experts was convened and eventually issued a series of recommendations that were formulated into legislation or executive action. Among the most noteworthy were (a) the attempts to develop community programs though the expansion of community mental health centers; (b) the creation of the National Institute of Child Health and Human Development, which included a mental retardation research branch; and (c) direct legislation P.L. 88-164, the Mental Retardation Services and Community Mental Health Center Construction Act. As shown in Table 6.1, along with a description of other key legislation for the mentally retarded and developmentally disabled, P.L. 88-164 was aimed at involving universities in research, training, and program development activities to advance the state of the art in the field, improve the quality of personnel and, in doing so, foster the development of new leadership and provide the impetus for the creation of innovative programs, esecially those based in the community. The direct immediate result of P.L. 88-164 was the creation of the Mental Retardation Research Centers and University Affiliated Facilities. An ongoing university-based professional constituency was created with a commitment to and vested interest in assuring that funds for research, training, and services for the mentally retarded continued to flow at a satisfactory level.

THE POST-KENNEDY ERA

The era of hope and action that began with the Kennedy administration continued in the years that followed. President Lyndon B. Johnson made the President's Panel on Mental Retardation into a permanent presidential advisory group, the President's Committee on Mental Retardation (PCMR). As an agent to promote change, PCMR still performs advisory, advocacy, and public information functions, both within and outside of government. Several PCMR publications, including *Changing Patterns of Residential Care for the Mentally Retarded,* published in 1969 and revised in 1976, the 1976 *Century of Decision* series and the 1980 *Mental Retardation: The Leading Edge—Service Programs That Work,* all had significant impact in promoting community care.

By the late 1960s, a growing and increasingly vocal constituency for change had emerged to whom local, state, and federal legislators and other elected officials had to pay attention. When not advocating for legislative change, the constituents pressed mental hygiene officials for improvements in services, deinstitutionalization, community residence development, preschool programs, adult services, and more and better special educational programs. Representatives of consumer groups pressed state legislatures for and achieved removal of mental retardation services from the psychiatric domination of the mental hygiene system.

These lobbying efforts led to substantial administrative reorganization. In several states, Offices or Departments of Mental Retardation were established with separate commissioners in charge of these executive components of state governments. While in most states psychiatrists maintained their domination of Departments of Mental Health, in some states controversy ensued over appointments to the directorships of the new Offices or Departments of Mental Retardation (and Developmental Disabilities). Openly competitive, professionals within or outside these systems vied for these positions with each other and with individuals, occasionally consumers, who were experienced in working for a voluntary agency or who had a background in public administration, especially if the latter individuals had fiscal expertise.

Ascent to leadership positions in the mental retardation field could, therefore, be achieved by progress on several different possible career tracks. The first group were professionals who "grew up" within the system and gained higher-level positions through their expertise. Direct personal relationships with political figures also helped. Most of the current generation of these leaders were trained as psychologists, social workers or special educators.

A second group of leaders, either with an administrative background and/or professional training, evolved from the voluntary sector of nonprofit agencies who have been a growing force in service provision in several states. Some of these agency leaders were themselves parents of a handicapped child and were therefore viewed by political leaders as being somewhat immune from criticism that they were indifferent to the plight of the mentally retarded. This judgment did not always prove correct, since these individuals soon became the "targets" when they were held responsible for the inadequacies of the systems they directed.

The third route to leadership appears to arise from individuals who could be considered "professional administrators" or technocrats. They often have experience running a department in state government, and are familiar with fiscal and/or administrative aspects of working in a state system and are capable of dealing with political issues.

Selection of administrative leadership also began to reflect the political bent of the leadership of the state government; i.e., whether the governor preferred a charismatic leader, who usually had a reformist bent and intended to change, improve, or dismantle an institutional system, or one more conservative in nature, merely intended to administer or manage an institutional system without significant attempts to change it.

Lobbying

In order to promote the desired change in the institutional system and the development of alternative programs in the community, consumers or their representative organizations began to lobby systematically for legislative actions. Only when traditional lobbying efforts failed to correct perceived injustices, or when frustrated by the slow pace of change, did these groups seek legal help, usually allying themselves with civil liberties groups that brought class action law suits against institutions or states.

An interesting phenomenon relating to the growth of consumer political activism for the mentally retarded was the extent that it stimulated other groups concerned with the developmentally disabled to, first, seek inclusion of the special disablity group they represented into what was initially legislation for the mentally retarded and, subsequently, to join in coalitions to effect changes for all handicapped individuals. The original Mental Retardation Facilities and Construction Act, P.L. 88-164, was passed in 1963 after considerable input from mental retardation professionals and knowledgeable consumers. When other disability groups became aware of the importance of the legislation, and realized that funding for future programs could be dependent upon being specifically denoted in future legislation, they pressed for a change in the original act. The result was a modification of the original legislation, P.L. 91-517, passed in 1970 and titled the Developmental Disabilities (D.D.) Facilities and Construction act. Disabilities such as cerebral palsy, epilepsy, and related neurological disorders were added to mental retardation as conditions covered by the act. P.L. 91-517 defined the term "developmental disability" as follows:

> A disability attributable to mental retardation, cerebral palsy, epilepsy, or another neurological condition of an individual found by the Secretary to be closely related to mental retardation or to require treatment similar to that required for mentally retarded individuals, which disability originates before such individual attains age eighteen, which has continued or can be expected to continue indefinitely, and which constitutes a substantial handicap to such individuals.

As Breen and Richman pointed out in Wiegerink and Pelosi's book on the D.D. movement, the definition clustered three categorical disorders: mental retardation, cerebral palsy, and epilepsy. Breen and Richman pointed out that it was important to understand the thinking of those who developed the definition since, in 1970, empirical data agreed on two points: (a) that all three of the conditions are major causes of substantial handicaps to adults disabled in childhood, and (b) that all three of the disorders imply multiple handicaps requiring special and similar services thoughout childhood and adult life.

In 1975, P.L. 94-103 was passed amending the D.D. act to become the Developmentally Disabled Assistance and Bill of Rights Act. Autism was added to the definition. But when contemplating the renewal of the Developmental Disabilities (D.D.) act as formulated in P.L. 94-103, Congress expressed concern about the definition of D.D. Legislators were under continuing pressure to add new disorders, and some objected to a "disease of the month or year" approach to defining needs within legislation. This was particularly disturbing since the thrust of the legislation otherwise appeared to be functional and noncategorical in intent. Finally, pressure also began to mount to add learning disabilities to the disorders covered. For these reasons, plus fear of offering a too open-ended definition that might expand eligibility not only under this act but also under other entitlement programs, Congress requested a study of the definition of D.D. The Department of Health, Education and Welfare responded by commissioning such a study.

Conducted by a private consulting group but with an advisory panel that included representatives from a broad range of interests in the D.D. field, the final recommendation of the study panel was a change to a functional definition that would be comprehensive but emphasize the severe and lasting nature of the disability. A strong dissenting minority opinion among panelists urged retention of a mention of specific disabilities. Others rejected the functional definition out of concern that individuals with milder disabilities but still in need would be unfairly excluded.

With some minor modifications the panel's newly recommended definition was incorporated into the 1978 revision of the law. The Title I Amendments to the P.L. 95-602, part of the Section titled Services and Facilities for the Mentally Retarded and Persons With Other Developmental Disabilities, Sec. 102 (7) defined developmental disability as:

> A severe, chronic disability of a person which –(A) is attributable to a mental or physical impairment or combination of mental and physical impairments; (B) is manifested before the person attains the age twenty-two; (C) is likely to continue indefinitely; (D) results in substantial functional limitations in three or more of the following areas of major life activity: (i) self-care, (ii) receptive and expressive language, (iii) learning, (iv) mobility, (v) self-direction, (vi) capacity for independent living, and (vii) economic sufficiency; and (E) reflects the person's need for a combination and sequence of special interdisciplinary, or generic care, treatment, or other services which are of life-long or extended duration and are individually planned and coordinated.

The impact of the new modified definition remains unclear, although a follow-up study group, in a report to Congress in January 1981, indicated that the change in the definition has had little overall impact. Despite the committee's language accompanying the act, indicating Congress's intent that disabilities previously included in the act should continue to be covered, fears persist that the new definition could be used to exclude individuals from services. Thus far, these worries have not been justified. Nevertheless, consumer groups and advocates remain vigilant to assure that cutbacks in services are not the result of semantic changes that may lend themselves to adverse bureaucratic interpretations.

The 1970 act, P.L. 91-517, had one other significant addition, the creation of planning and advisory councils that included input from consumer representatives. The 1975 D.D. act, P.L. 94-103, required both consumer and professional membership, including mandated state governmental representation. The councils were instructed to develop long-range plans for state developmental disability services and to continue their responsibility for determining the use of federal funds allocated in the act as a formula grant program for developmental disability services.

The 1975 act, P.L. 94-103, added two key provisions. The first was the creation of a Protection and Advocacy (P and A) Agency for each participating state. The second was the addition of a Bill of Rights provision that attempted to set legal minimum standards for services in facilities receiving federal funds

In working to renew this legislation or expand it, a coalition formed that eventually included representatives of almost every group concerned with developmental disabilities, including consumer organizations, directors of state programs, University Affiliated Facilities, Developmental Disablity Councils, and Protection and Advocacy agencies. As a result, until recently these groups were successful in assuring a steady growth of funds allocated for the D.D. act's three major activities: the UAFs, the D.D. Council–administered formula grant programs, and the P and A agencies. The strength of these constituent groups in maintaining the provisions in the Developmental Disabilities Act is illustrated by the successful opposition to the recent thrust to eliminate the D.D. act and to include the elements in block grants to the states. The D.D. act was not only kept intact, but administration attempts at achieving funding reductions were largely unsuccessful.

The political power of the mental retardation and developmental disability group is formidable. State D.D. Council and P and A agencies are present in almost every state. Members of D.D. Councils are usually political appointees, often with good political contacts or know-how. Protection and Advocacy agencies attract politically active lawyers or other advocates. University Affiliated Facilities, a prominent component of the act since its very beginning, are located in thirty-six states and represent a key tertiary referral source in their state and serve all social classes, including relatives of a number of legislators and elected officials. Many UAFs are key program, training, or research components of state universities and powerful private institutions of higher learning. Each element of the D.D. act receiving funding support under the provision of the act has potentially powerful connections throughout the country. Added to this constituency are the consumer groups with hundreds of thousands of members nationwide, representing a constituency of 6 to 10 million individuals, not all of whom may be voters, but whose families may be. They have important allies among legislators and politicians. Some, such as Senator Lowell Weicker, were or are themselves parents or relatives of a disabled child. Other strong legislative supporters, regardless of political affiliation, simply act out of deeply held convictions to help the handicapped. For example, Senator Jacob Javits, a liberal, developed and advocated for the Bill of Rights Section of the Developmental Disabilities Act, while Senator Orin Hatch, a conservative, also actively supported its continuation. The same combination of consumer advocacy and concerned legislators was productive in bringing about many progressive changes on state and local levels.

Recent Rehabilitation and Education Legislation

In the past decade, very important legislation was passed to remove the physical barriers that prevented access to public facilities, as well as the bureaucratic or attitudinal barriers to needed programs. While the mental retardation and developmental disabilities advocates were always concerned about rehabilitation programs, vocational training, and physical barriers to facilities, their efforts to extend these benefits to the more severely handicapped population among their constituency began to bear fruit only in the 1970s. The Rehabilitation Act of 1973, P.L. 93-112, represented a legislative milestone, encouraging the inclusion of severely retarded individuals in vocational training programs. With the added incentive of some federal financial support for states, this act also included a powerful provision in the celebrated Section 504 which, once administrative regulations were approved in 1977, demanded equal access for all handicapped individuals to public facilities and programs receiving federal support.

It also became evident in the 1970s that existing special education programs did not meet the needs of mentally retarded and developmentally disabled children. States and localities had too few programs, and many that existed were inadequate. Therefore, political pressure mounted from both consumer and professional groups to upgrade and expand special educational services. This effort led to the 1975 passage of what must be considered momentous legislation, P.L. 94-142, the Education for All Handicapped Children Act, which insisted upon access to free public education for all school age handicapped children, regardless of type or degree of disability. It also provided some limited incentives to encourage preschool program development.

Although the fiscal incentives, now amounting to about 1.2 billion dollars, for the states were not high, P.L. 94-142 spurred states to expand their service commitment to handicapped children. A more democratic process was established to decide what programs should be offered to a particular child. The number of children attending special education programs grew rapidly, and the quality of programs generally improved. The implementation of P.L. 94-142 has not always gone smoothly; some states and localities grumble about the limited federal support that accompanied the strenuous demands and requirements of the law, and others complain about the competition for limited resources between handicapped children and their nonhandicapped peers, or about the serious problems in coordinating or providing related services. Nonetheless, an important result of P.L. 94-142 is its high level of acceptance by professionals, consumers, and the public of the handicapped child's right to education and the opening of the school door to many who, in the past, had had no opportunity to attend a school program. (Chapter 7 gives a detailed discussion of the rights of handicapped children to education under P.L. 94-142.)

Political Issues in Funding, Health, and Residential Care

While universal health insurance has been a potent and controversial item on the American political agenda since it was introduced by President Truman in the post–World War II period, its antecedents are the Social Security laws of the 1930s that provided income for the unemployed and the disabled. Not until the 1964 passage of Medicare (the Title XVIII Amendments to the Social Security Act) did government-supported health care for a finite population, the elderly, become a reality. This milestone in welfare legislation, which may be viewed as a comprehensive insurance program or as a form of insurance against catastrophe for a population with a high risk of suffering from a costly acute or chronic disability, was the beginning of an expanding federal support for the care of the chronically handicapped. Another important step was the passage of Title XIX, originally intended to provide care for the poor or the medically indigent, but expanded by the Nixon administration to assume chronic care costs through the Intermediate Care Facility program, a mechanism seized upon by the states to cover the costs of their institutional care systems for the mentally retarded.

With the sizable and growing elderly population in the United States, it is not hard to understand the political pressures that resulted in the Medicare legalization. Yet the political forces behind the passage of Title XIX and its amendment to serve the residential populations in institutions appear more subtle. It represented the combined efforts of those striving to help the poor and then the disabled to obtain improved health care, and the contrasting interests of legislators and elected officials attempting to relieve both private and municipal hospitals, as well as state governments operating costly residential care facilities, of the financial burden in providing acute and chronic care for the indigent and handicapped populations. The subsequent pressures to extend the Title XIX program to reimburse for care provided in community facilities was seen as a mechanism to fund deinstitutionalization efforts. While this extention of support was initially welcomed by both state officials and consumer representatives, it was subsequently seriously questioned by advocates as leading to a programmatically restrictive or unwanted "medical model" for community care.

It should also be noted that, in some states, Title XX of the Social Security Act, an initially open-ended mechanism for the states to offset social service costs, was also used to finance community residential care. Federal fiscal pressures resulted in capping the expenditures from this legislation, however, and then eventually incorporated this provision in a block grant, which further limited the availability of funds as a source for community residential care.

The role of the judiciary in the development of community programs for the mentally retarded must also be noted. Class action law suits have led to court judgments spurring the development of community residences; and courts have also struck down attempts to use zoning regulations to restrict the use of single-family homes for group residences in some communities.

RECENT POLITICAL FRICTIONS

With the acceleration of deinstitutionalization in the 1970s and the creation of alternative programs in the community, frictions and controversies of a political nature were inevitable. The involvement of the media in the early 1970s—with exposés of the evils of institutions, as in the Willowbrook case—created a politically charged atmosphere in which state legislatures, state executives, commissioners, and high-level institutional personnel sought out scapegoats to blame for the inhumane conditions and untoward events. A rapid change in personnel followed in some institutions as well as in positions at a commissioner's level. At the same time, the exposés, and the court suits that often followed, provided the leverage needed by advocates to force governors and state legislatures to appropriate more funds to upgrade institutional care and/or create community alternatives.

At the same time, the attacks on institutions and the dispersion of their residents created political tensions, mainly around job-related issues. Many large institutions located in rural communities are a major source of employment; a phase-down or closing has adverse effects on the area's economy and is an obvious source of concern to local politicians. This is one reason why there is usually strong legislative opposition to closing facilities. Furthermore, civil service employee unions oppose the resultant layoffs of state workers, particularly when the alternative is a state contract with a voluntary or private agency to operate both the community-based residential services and the required support services. Since lower-paid nonunion workers often replace public service employees, considerable pressure has been mounted, both at state and federal levels, to retrain institutional employees for community positions and/or to avoid layoffs. Some disruption and job loss will always occur, since the exodus of institutional residents to their home communities may create jobs too far distant from where the institutional employees now live. Without serious retraining, the interests of lower-level staff are unprotected, and their representatives continue to present an obstacle to deinstitutionalization.

Other vested interests also oppose deinstitutionalization. The bureaucrats in administrative positions (e.g., food and clothing purchasing and delivery), as well as the suppliers of these goods, fear the dissolution of institutions and diffusion of residents to community sites where the buying of goods will be from many local merchants. Therefore, major contractors to state facilities, and perhaps even builders or construction unions involved with building or renovating large facilities, may lobby against the dissolution of the institutional system.

Resistance to community residence development and the deinstitutionalization process also comes from local communities, who often oppose group homes within their midst. They fear negative effects on property values, a change in the character of neighborhoods, and the disabled strangers living or the staff working in these residences (with the opposition sometimes having racial overtones). Homeowners in these neighborhoods contact their local legislators, only a minority of whom assume pro-community residence positions, and most of whom side with the opponents or attempt to remain aloof from the controversy. The organized opposition generated by the controversies makes it even more difficult for state legislatures to expand appropriations for community residences.

As a consequence of this process of site selection, communities have demanded greater control over the choice of locations for community residences. This demand was followed by site selection legislation which, for example, in New York requires a deadline for local reactions to the establishment of a community residence, once the residential site is officially considered by the state Office of Mental Retardation and Developmental Disabilities. An appeals procedure was built in to deal with dissatisfaction in the community. Unfortunately, communities have found many means to evade the process or circumvent the law, such as arranging for private purchase of potential sites or attempting to intimidate the seller so he or she will not do business with the state. As an alternative, it is not surprising that some private enterprises and parent-founded voluntary agencies have taken direct responsibility for providing community care. Noteworthy is the fact that, with the expansion of voluntary or private agency operation of group residences, these agencies become another involved party advocating for the establishment of these community residences. Unfortunately, community opposition appears almost as great to facilities operated by voluntary agencies as to those proposed to be operated by a state agency. Once community residences are established and in place, community acceptance appears to grow, although saturation of areas with several residences has been a related political problem.

An interesting facet to the involvement of voluntary agencies in the provision of community care, either residential or day program, is that, once the facilities are opened, the voluntary agencies become mutually interdependent partners to the state agency. The voluntary sector tends to lobby legislatures to assure continuation of adequate funding for the residences they operate and, in doing so, perform an advocacy function that the state agency itself is not in a tenable position to perform.

Recently the schism has widened between advocates of community care and those working to preserve the institutions. It has been proposed that ICF-MR (Title XIX) funding supporting institutional care be terminated in seven to ten years, forcing the conversion of the federal funds supporting institutional care into use for community care. Those opposing this radical legislative proposal point to its potentially negative sequellae, including disruptions to the operations of facilities and the probable adverse effects on residents. Furthermore, failure to meet early deinstitutionalization target dates mandated by court decrees has occurred repeatedly. Another growing concern is that potential conflicts will be aggravated between a privileged institutional class of clients who can carry their ICF dollars back with them into the community, and the never-institutionalized population, who have no such funding support or access to care. Finally, it must be pointed out that, before an effective community care system can be developed, a "front loading" of funds is required to create a critical mass or network of basic community programs, staffed by well-trained individuals, all of which are necessary to sustain any massive community placement effort.

It is hard to predict how the struggle between contending points of view will be resolved. The trend toward community care will probably continue as long as the movement engenders sufficient political support. The extent of this support will depend upon whether community care is viewed as economical, and of high quality, and, finally, upon the strength of the constituency supporting the community care movement.

7

Legal Rights of Dependent Persons

The decade of the 1970s saw the broad affirmation of the human rights of the disabled. 1981 was the International Year of Disabled Persons, and reminded us how far we still have to go in realizing internationally recognized declarations of rights. Despite a broad affirmation of fundamental human rights, machinery has not been established for giving them effective legal protection. Remedies are required to support these rights.

Comprehensive community services require access to the justice system. Ensuring access to the justice system involves, among other things, rules changes, opportunities for representation, and the availability of judicial and nonjudicial forums for dispute resolution. Most disputes do not have to involve the courts. For some mentally retarded or developmentally disabled persons, however, problems of access are compounded by custodial confinement, geographic isolation, and the individual's (or the family's) difficulties in identifying a problem as "legal," that is, knowing when statutory rights have been violated. Even when a clear sense of injustice is present, a family or an individual may have difficulty locating, retaining, or guiding a lawyer or trained lay advocate.

Until the 1970s the legal profession, for the most part, ignored the rights of mentally retarded and other handicapped persons. The situation has changed rapidly in the past decade. Federal and state legislation, judicial opinions and public policy pronouncements, as well as consumer organizations, advocacy groups, and professional associations, have all contributed to new expectations and have made new demands on our judicial system.

The Right to Education

A NEW DEAL FOR HANDICAPPED CHILDREN

Enacted in 1975, the Education for All Handicapped Children Act (Public Law 94-142) has been implemented in some form in every school district in the United States. This regulation makes it clear that all handicapped children will, by law, be assured of a "free, appropriate public education." These words understate the full impact of the intent of the legislation. Its specific features were designed to produce sweeping changes in special education, creating mechanisms for finding and identifying handicapped children, creating individualized educational programs for them, and educating them in a nondiscriminatory way in the least restrictive, appropriate environment. Maximum feasible participation in planning by parents and teachers is required. Deciding on the educational plan is to be a process involving the child's parents and the child (where appropriate) as well as school personnel; parents are to be notified and given fair hearings when they do not agree with school personnel on programs for their child; and staff involved in educating handicapped children are to be appropriately trained for this task. The Education for All Handicapped Children's Act is a law that mandates education *and* civil rights for its beneficiaries at the same time. It is a powerful factor in securing the right to education, because it articulates national policy goals and outlines specific steps for local school districts to undertake to accomplish these goals.

This federal mandate is backed up in many states by education law and regulations of the commissioners of education. Sometimes these statues were in place before P.L. 94-142, and comprehensive services were required. Compliance, however, was made even less discretionary with the presence of the national policy embedded in federal law.

P.L. 94-142 can best be described as a comprehensive law, since it assumes that all services for handicapped children must be created *de novo*. Unless already deemed to be in place, all local school districts must create a plan to identify, locate, and evaluate all children in need of special education. These activities include in-school screening efforts involving informal and formal procedures and media campaigns designed to alert the general public to the needs and rights of handicapped children. Out-of-school children, even preschoolers, are considered prime candidates for attention.

Even when a child is identified, parents must receive written notice of recommended evaluations or placements of children suspected of having handicapping conditions. Included in notification to parents is a communication about their rights, and parents' consent must be obtained before the child undergoes any initial evaluation or is placed in a program. Since parents and children may feel stigmatized by labels that identify a child as handicapped, or by the educational program to which the child is assigned, these parent notice and consent procedures are designed to protect the rights of children and their parents in decisions regarding special education. The transmission of information from school personnel to parents is also intended to maximize parental involvement in the evaluation process and programming activities, and represents a key commitment of the writers of the law to school-family cooperation.

To prevent misclassification and false labeling, a multidisciplinary team evaluates the children suspected of having a handicapping condition. Moreover, the diagnostic procedures specified in the law will not permit the use of a single test score or procedure as the only measure considered in making a special education placement. The multidisciplinary team is composed of persons who know the child, the significance of the educational and other measurements taken on the child, and the programs available. Finally, all children receiving special education must be reevaluated every three years. School districts also have the responsibility to create a mechanism for dealing with disagreements between parents and school staff regarding evaluation and placement decisions. Parents or guardians of handicapped children are legally entitled to an impartial hearing and the right of appeal.

Before placement in special education takes place, each child must have a written individualized educational plan (IEP). Ideally, the IEP is the product of a working conference in which school staff, the child's parents, and the child (if appropriate) participate. This agreed-upon plan and program must include:

1. a statement of the child's present levels of educational performance;
2. a statement of annual goals, including short-term instructional objectives;
3. a statement of the specific special education and related services to be provided to the child, and the extent to which the child will be able to participate in regular educational programs;
4. the projected dates for initiation of services and the anticipated duration of the services; and
5. appropriate objective criteria and evaluation procedures and schedules for determining, at least on an annual basis, whether the short-term instructional objectives are being achieved (sections 330a, 346).

Since the changes encompassed by P.L. 94-142 were so comprehensive, the lawmakers recognized that local school districts could not carry out the intent of the act without familiarity with its statutes and retraining to produce qualified personnel. Each state therefore must plan and implement staff development, including in-service training of district and school personnel and the creation of new roles.

STATE GOVERNMENT AND P.L. 94-142

Among the most significant requirements imposed on the states by P.L. 94-142 is education for all handicapped persons between the ages of three and twenty-one. Moreover, the states must make sure that they service children previously unserved before improving existing programs, and must improve services to children where existing programs were below standards. In addition, since some handicapped children already receive educational services in state-operated facilities and some new and/or improved services must be started in these facilities, the state education departments became responsible under this law for supervising these services.

The state education departments are now also responsible for overseeing the local school districts: whether they are eligible to receive federal funds, whether nondiscriminatory testing of children takes place, and whether they guarantee due process under the law for children and their parents.

Finally, through a complex funding formula, federal, state, and local funds are now used to generate services that previously did not exist. With these incentives, improvements in some service areas provide a legislative remedy where the educational rights of children had been denied.

To some extent, this new federal law caught up to the state of the art. When P.L. 94-142 was passed, several states were administering special education under regulations that were substantially similar to those of the new federal legislation. These states were faced with the complex problem of restructuring special education according to the P.L. 94-142's specific guidelines, as opposed to the simpler task of fully adopting federal policy in the delivery of education to the handicapped.

The Protection of the Courts

Even before the development of legislation to protect the educational rights of the disabled, a number of major court decisions established the rights of the dependent population to protection from unsafe facilities and dangerous custodial practices. As in the celebrated Willowbrook case, several class action law suits have led to court judgments against state officials or agencies; and consent decrees and court approved plans were issued to protect institutional residents from harm.

Protection from harm meant adequate care, including the right to some forms of treatment and education. Specifications of these procedures called for the employment of qualified professionals to design and carry out treatment, with appropriate staff-client ratios. In the *Wyatt* v. *Stickney* decision, similar goals and procedures were specified, approaching a clear right to treatment philosophy. The long march out of the institutions and into community care was not initiated, but was certainly accelerated by these decisions.

These interventions by the courts have been accomplished despite the considered judgments and the opposition of professionals in the various states. Consequently, the courts have been criticized for being overzealous in setting unrealistic goals for deinstitutionalization and for attempting to operate facilities through court appointed review panels or masters. Higher-court rulings have recently been more guarded in calling for the rights of persons in custodial care to treatment, particularly in optimal settings. In the *Pennhurst* case, the Supreme Court emphasized the rights of residents to improved care and treatment, but refused to apply the civil rights components of P.L. 94-103 (see Table 6.1) to this institutional population. The court also hesitated to accept the judgment of outside professionals over state employed experts. In other words, when professional opinion differed, the court confessed uncertainty over what constitutes optimal treatment.

A similar retreat from involvement in professional controversies is evident in a recent decision in the *Willowbrook* case. The Appellate Court in

New York overturned the district court judge, who had ruled in favor of small, community-based facilities as the preferred location for resettlement from a large state facility. In other words, the Appellate Court questioned the need for small facilities of less than fifteen beds, once again citing differences in professional judgment as the reason for not decreeing a uniform standard of care. Despite a more conservative Supreme Court and other judiciaries, the basic underpinnings and philosophy for establishing the legal rights of the mentally retarded were set down in the decade of the 1970s.

Legal Rights and Advocacy

The expectation of full human rights for mentally retarded and developmentally disabled persons is emphasized in three developments. First, retarded people, like all others in society, are acknowledged to have definable legal and human rights. Second, older views that permitted the summary divestment of human and legal rights, on the basis of labeling and generalized assumptions of incompetency, are rejected. Third and perhaps most important, organized society has taken the first step to increase the probability that all disabled people will actually enjoy and exercise their legal rights.

The most important challenge of this decade is to realize the legal rights that protect dependent persons. Although litigation, especially "impact case" judgments (e.g., test cases, class action law suits), remains a major tool for access to justice, there is increasing recognition that alternative forums, such as administrative hearings, human rights committees, and other mechanisms for handling complaints, are also needed to secure access to speedy and efficient remedies. Consumers, the advocacy movement, and self-advocates should continue to press for the establishment of effective grievance procedures in residential care or other service settings.

Advocacy needs and possibilities have expanded rapidly through major litigative and legislative advances. In the wake of *Mills* and *PARC*, as well as other court decisions that recognize the retarded child's right to education, Congress has created new means of legal advocacy on behalf of all handicapped children within the educational process. Further, court decisions establishing the right to treatment, habilitation, and "protection from harm" have often led to additional or improved access to due process. Examples are the challenges that have emerged dealing with the adequacy and restrictiveness of residential placements. Finally, revised state codes and regulations, as well as Medicaid regulations, have set out a wide panoply of rights for those who are already eligible for state-provided services.

Congress has also moved to increase the prospect of disabled persons obtaining their rights in 24-hour care settings. The U. S. Department of Justice now has the authority to negotiate and/or litigate "where there is a pattern of resistance to the full enjoyment" of the institutionalized person's constitutional and federal statutory rights. Symbolically and practically, passage of the Rights of Institutionalized Persons Act is a significant advance, but this law must be implemented through a program of vigorous investigation, remediation, and enforcement. Does the Justice Department have a sufficiently large legal and paralegal staff to secure these rights? Further, as the various dependent populations covered by this act move from state-run facilities to private nursing homes and board-and-care residences, other steps must be taken to avoid merely shifting the location of the abuses. Congress incorporated such an assumption in the expectation that states can and will monitor these facilities.

Even with adequate allocations of personnel, the Justice Department can handle only the most blatant complaints. Legally established advocacy systems must be able to assist residents in community facilities and those living in their own homes, as well as having the authority to seek remedies for vulnerable residents. Protection and advocacy systems (P and A), Legal Services Corporation programs, and other local advocates are often in a better position to effect a speedy and locally relevant remedy than more-distant branches of other law enforcement agencies. Without an ongoing system of client-oriented advocacy, it will be difficult to promote and monitor the quality of community-based services, accountability to clients, and respect for the legal and human rights of the mentally retarded and the developmentally disabled. Experience shows that advocates working on sustained local, state, and national levels are key components in making rights a reality.

Yet implementation of programs to protect the legal rights of dependent persons can lag behind statutory enactments. In 1978, for example, the District of Columbia adopted a new code with stringent procedural safeguards and a clear statutory right to both legal counsel and lay advocacy; yet these advocacy provisions are not in place, and considerable citizen pressure has proved necessary to secure the funding for implementing this reform statute. The various states have also varied greatly in the extent to which they have provided funds for client-oriented advocacy. Underfunding has limited the supervision of guardianship, commitment, and residential placement laws, and the way in which such laws are administered. The Michigan Association for Retarded Citizens brought suit against state officials for trivializing the guardianship process, a determination that can make a major difference in the life of a mentally retarded individual. In a striking example of assembly line processing, the association documented that the state granted 100 petitions in eighty minutes, all without benefit of an advocate or an individualized inquiry.

In general, the support for quality advocacy has been woefully limited. Massachusetts, for example, a recent survey found, annually spent only two cents per person for state-funded mental disability advocacy. In contrast, Michigan spent four times, New Jersey six times, New York ten times, Vermont twelve times, and Illinois sixteen times as much per capita. While it is certainly necessary that P and A systems be adequately funded by governmental agencies to remedy this scarcity of advocates, generic legal services providers, such as legal aid organizations, Bar Associations, and other public interest groups must also increase their activities on behalf of this sorely underserved population.

In addition, more public information is needed on how various grievance settling programs and oversight mechanisms work. Are human rights committees in agencies a common or isolated phenomenon? What characteristics of such committees are associated with effective functioning, and what characteristics are associated with poor performance? Are there differences in the performance of oversight bodies that derive from courts, legislatures, or departmental regulation? What types of complaints do they receive, and how are they handled? How should human rights committees relate to statewide ombudsman agencies and client-oriented advocacy organizations? Do these procedures and organizations increase respect for the rights of clients among service providers?

It is ironic that advocacy for the mentally retarded has led to the arbitrary creation of different classes of citizens, each with different entitlements to services. For example, successful class action lawsuits have given the Willowbrook population access to funding and services which their peers, who are equally deserving, but without any history of having been institutionalized, cannot obtain. It is probable that legal action will be attempted in the rest of the 1980s to redress this imbalance in rights and access to services.

This inequity can be a particularly bothersome impediment in the development of community services, whereas *Willowbrook*, *Partlow* and other early court cases emphasized upgrading of care in a large deficient facility. Depopulation has indeed proceeded apace in these facilities, but so has the increase in per capita expenditure on those who remain institutionalized. The complicity of the Health Care Financing Administration in this trend must be noted, but a share of blame should also rest with Congress. By "capping" funds in 1972 for social services, the most adaptable mechanism for staffing small residences and various day services, Congress placed increased pressure on the open-ended "health-related" funding streams. Individuals who have always lived in the community or with their families are particularly penalized by the loss of support for social service funding for respite care, day care, homemaker services, early intervention, case management, and protective services.

The challenge of the 1980s is to create a society that will fully respect the rights of persons with developmental disabilities and welcome their participation as integrated members. In part, this will require a rationalized, nationwide standard of legal protection so that entitlements do not depend on the accident of place of residence or the ability to mount a successful class action lawsuit. At one level, this means examining outmoded funding formulae and legislation that perpetuate discrimination and impede access to the services of choice. At a more basic level, better ways must be found to respect people's choice-making capacities and to resolve as many complaints as possible through accessible and nonintimidating advocacy forums. This country continues to prize the citizen's right to a day in court, but it must also take steps to ensure access to effective channels to help those long denied the means of presenting complaints and redressing grievances.

8

Staffing and Training

The recruitment and training of personnel to provide community services to the mentally retarded assumes that such persons require knowledge of the client population, their needs and expectations, and an understanding of the settings and systems of which they are a part. Whether service providers are employees of a voluntary agency or a state-supported facility, their orientation will need to include information on how to work with clients who have a life-long disorder and with other professionals and nonprofessionals involved in the provision of integrated services. Programmatically, such understanding includes both the fundamental tasks to be performed and the responsibility that agencies and employees bear for the health and safety of clients. While training must include the specifics of the job, other aspects should not be ignored. These generally encompass an introduction to the agency, an understanding of mental retardation and related developmental disabilities, the planning of services, and the techniques required in effective case management. A model curriculum might include such topics as individual job expectations, exceptional support and situations, normal development, and observational skills. Under this training mandate the employee can begin to learn to negotiate the system, to begin to team up with others. Communication skills thereby become one of the central foci of training; an interdisciplinary setting becomes the optimal situation or environment in which this can occur.

Practical experience is a necessary component of all training and is generally rendered through supervised clinical exposure in existing programs. In these settings, community care workers probably receive "hands on" training with supervision during the first few weeks or months of employment. An optimal situation involves the assignment of a fellow worker to acquaint the newcomer with the role expectations and procedures of service delivery. Both partners in this kind of learning situation have found this experience worthwhile.

The key to effective and comprehensive community services is the availability of a productive staff who are properly trained and supervised. Traditional institutions and new residential alternatives, such as privately operated ICF-MRs, have had difficulties retaining such personnel. Even those staff who stay in direct care positions often perform their roles in a disinterested and uninvolved way. This situation may be attributed to a number of factors, of which lack of opportunity for advancement, poor role models (i.e., inadequate or inappropriate supervision), and low pay scales are of greatest importance. For example, in 42 percent of group homes in the state of Washington, turnover rates of 100 percent have been reported. Moreover, in a recent survey of more than 2,000 administrators of private residential programs, 84 percent of the respondents cited recruitment, training, and retention of staff as major problems.

The most serious factor leading to high turnover seems to be the economic one. Sixteen randomly selected public institutions with annual turnover rates of 50 percent or higher were compared with sixteen facilities having rates 15 percent or lower. Employees in institutions with the highest turnover indicated an average starting salary $1,500 lower than those with less turnover. In addition to the lack of pay incentive, most residential facilities offer limited opportunity for advancement. A hidden factor involves job satisfaction: employees feel they have little or no autonomy, i.e., they have no role in the decision-making process.

A related problem is that salaries in voluntary, agency-operated community residences are far lower than those received by service workers in large, traditional, state institutions. Some claim that the work is more demanding in large traditional institutions housing more severely disabled persons. Nevertheless community service personnel may be more visible and have considerably greater responsibility; their work is no less stressful; and they are faced with many of the same problems.

Turnover may be remedied by rationalizing the pay of employees and restructuring the job ladder to provide upgrading opportunities not based solely on educational attainment. The issue, however, cannot be as narrowly defined in dealing with job satisfaction and autonomy. Decentralization of services, with its accompanying divestment of central control, can potentially increase staff decision-making, permitting managers of smaller facilities to allow their personnel in that unit to set their own priorities. With programs in thirty-six states, technical assistance to support the introduction of such models can be obtained from many of the federally funded University Affiliated Facilities or programs (UAFs). The UAFs have trained professionals and nonprofessionals over the last sixteen years; many of these UAFs have developed curricula and have trained others who have themselves become trainers of direct care personnel. In short, the University Affiliated Facilities can serve as a resource for preparing community staff in the delivery of more diversified services that are more closely articulated with their own neighborhoods and communities.

Reconceptualizing the Caring Function

Basic organizational research pinpoints the need to look at systemwide conditions encouraging unproductive performance. In particular, many persons employed in providing residential services for the mentally retarded perceive themselves as powerless—even as victimized—as the clients they serve. The organizational environment is not responsive to their need for autonomy at work and in the marketplace; in short, they see their role as lacking in meaningful involvement and not allowing them to become self-actualized.

The jobs such people perform are often seen by others as unimportant and as requiring little skill. Within the system the care-giving staff is ranked somewhere near the bottom; perhaps for this reason they are not encouraged to talk about their work, express ideas, nor offer suggestions. Seldom solicited for their observations about residents, the care givers have little to say about the formation or implementation of policy affecting themselves or the people for whom they care. Support for this view is offered by Raynes, Pratt, and Roses in their study of a large public institution.

> The provision of resident-stimulating care is positively related to the extent to which direct-care staff, both the people in charge of the buildings and the aides working with them, perceive themselves to be involved in making decisions relating to their work and the residents in their care.

The stress of providing 24-hour-a-day care can be reduced by sharing other tasks, such as representing the unit at meetings and program planning. More important, it can provide people with a sense of accomplishment, particularly if there is opportunity to review their progress. Client progress evaluation can help employees recognize their own accomplishments, provided it is not used to assess an employee's effectiveness, since client variables make this an inaccurate gauge of relative performance by staff members with differing responsibilities. By providing the staff with a simple means of evaluating the client's progress, positive effects on job satisfaction are obtained.

If the staff is to be involved in the full dimension of the work at hand, they should be taught to measure client progress in regard to goals and objectives they are helping to formulate. Such a system of nonhierarchical evaluation requires that individual habilitation plans be designed and carried out in what may be called a "program unit," encompassing a relatively small group of clients and staff with a relatively low formal division of labor. In this kind of human service work organization, persons working at different levels in close interpersonal collaboration can help plan, carry out, and evaluate the functions of their unit.

A major source of employee dissatisfaction is lack of career opportunity for the experienced worker. Lakin and Bruininks suggest various ways of increasing promotional opportunities within the residential service system. Scholarships and/or release time for employees wishing to further their education may be provided, sometimes linked to a system that allows workers to acquire credits toward a degree for their on-the-job experience. It is also an incentive for employees to know that job promotions are available, since such promotions ensure that experienced staff are not lost to turnover.

When job retention rates increase, less time is spent on recruitment and training, and personnel responsible for staff training can spend more time on providing in-service training. Promotion from within can be linked directly to employees' level of skill. In sum, a dynamic system is dependent in some measure on the opportunity it offers its employees for advancement.

Retraining Institutional Personnel

While turnover and work dissatisfaction are major problems, many loyal and skilled public service workers are threatened with job loss as a result of deinstitutionalization. The effort to close down traditional institutions has left many states with an obligation to retrain direct care staff for community residential and support services. Many of the promises made to these employees, who are often protected by state civil service statutes, have not been fulfilled. Changes in Pennsylvania and New York, for example, recommended relocation of institutional personnel into community settings, with compensation to be provided by the state government. According to this plan, employees could also have the option of transferring within the state system. The retraining for support of such transfers was limited, and the transfers were a "one-way street": employees could not come back. In New York, employees were encouraged to qualify for higher-level civil service positions through education and training. Those unable to qualify, however, were not allowed to return to their former civil service ranking, and few employees opted to risk their tenure.

Federal legislation supporting job restructuring, training and upgrading for displaced public employees is on the books. Congress has mandated such protections in the Mental Health and Developmental Disabilities acts. The regulations governing the Developmental Disabilities Act, as amended by P.L. 95-602, require each state participating in the federally funded program to provide for the proper training and placement of former institutional employees in a community setting. Despite these federal mandates, training and career incentives for the vast majority of institutional employees have been quite limited.

In the main, program managers believe that former institutional employees can be useful in community settings, provided they receive the proper orientation and retraining. Some former institutional employees are rated as above-average foster family care providers. Furthermore, it has been reported that former institutional staff working toward changing the disruptive or aberrant behavior of a client are more patient than community workers who have less experience with this population.

Retrained institutional staff are goal-directed when employed in client-centered organizational environments. In a three-year effort to convert institutionally based services, the skills possessed by institutional direct care employees were virtually equivalent to those of community facility employees, and many, with the benefit of training related to values and orientation in community services plus appropriate supervision and support, possessed the competency needed for effective performance in community facilities.

Professional Personnel

Authorization for direct federal support for the training of professional personnel in the field is to be found under the Developmental Disablities Act, the Maternal and Child Health (MCH) legislation (Title V, Social Security Act and the recent MCH Block Grant), and the Education for All Handicapped Children Act of 1975. The Developmental Disabilities Act and successor legislation provided funds to university-based programs to offer interdisciplinary training to some nineteen professions working with handicapped persons.

Graduates of the Maternal and Child Health supported training programs, including thousands receiving interdisciplinary training over the past sixteen years at the UAF centers across the country, have had a significant role to play in the management and development of programs and in relevant research. As the mandates to reduce institutional populations and to carry out the provisions of P.L. 94-142 (Education for All Handicapped Children Act) are emphasized, the need for community programming will continue to grow. In this, the efforts of the UAF programs, with their special emphasis on interdisciplinary training will be of particular importance in meeting future manpower needs, particularly in providing leaders to ensure the success of the new programs.

Specifically, the success of training physicians in an interdisciplinary UAF setting, in this case under the mandate of the maternal and child health program, is illustrated by a survey of some forty-three physician-fellows trained at the Children's Evaluation and Rehabilitation Center, Rose F. Kennedy Center of the Albert Einstein College of Medicine. The followup report indicates that thirty-six assumed leadership roles in the field, while seven other professionals, educators, and psychologists are program directors in the voluntary sector. Similar results are reported by other UAFs, such as those at Johns Hopkins University and Children's Hospital in Boston.

Under the provision of P.L. 94-142, the states are mandated to develop and implement a comprehensive system of personnel development. To this end, the federal Office of Education, in its 1979 report, noted that it is critical that "teachers be trained to serve the most severely handicapped children since the law places the highest priority on serving this population." To meet this need, numerous in-service projects have been funded by this office. Part of this effort was an attempt to increase the number of special educators by linking the training to other programs already providing professional training. Some additional training was provided under contract with the UAFs (and others) by the Division of Personnel Preparation, Bureau for Education of the Handicapped. In all, 26,700 teachers received limited forms of in-service training in 1979. For special education teachers and related services combined, the numbers increased from 435,585 in school year 1979–80 to 440,109 in school year 1980–81. The bureau reiterates, however, that training of regular classroom teachers continues to be critical, and funds to facilitate training have been less readily available in the 1980s.

The clear trend is to provide for very young handicapped children, including those who benefited from regional neonatal intensive care units, so that they and their parents may receive timely services well before they reach elementary school age. This trend suggests the need for a policy to encourage the training of professionals to serve younger children. At the other end of the age spectrum, more retarded individuals are surviving, living longer, and requiring increased medical, residential, and social services. A significant "old age" population of elderly retarded, who require specialized services and appropriately trained staff to provide them, are coming to the attention of social service professionals. Professional development for the geriatic population needs to be increased before the problem gets out of hand.

The ability of agency providers to meet the need for high-quality comprehensive community services for people of all ages, of which education and residential care are two of the more significant services, will depend, in some measure, on satisfying their future manpower needs. A knowledge of the adaptive capacities of the target population provides an understanding of the requirements that should dictate the selection, training, and supervision of community service personnel.

In summary, professional personnel are needed to serve the preschool and school-aged child who is living at home or in a community facility. Effective case management personnel must be developed and trained to coordinate services and assist families to fulfill their goals, to manage the problems of retarded children and their families and of adults who are striving to achieve greater autonomy and self sufficiency than their counterparts in earlier generations.

Sound personnel planning should be future oriented. Tomorrow's shortages will not be the same as today's. Demographic and epidemiological data on community needs (such as the increasing number of retarded adults who are living in communities), service utilization data, present staffing patterns, occupational role performance measures, treatment outcome assessments, service cost data, and other factors also need to be considered to develop a comprehensive analysis of how best to fulfill the need for community service personnel.

9

Management and Accountability: Directing and Tracking a Community Service System

There are many definitions of what management does in the human service field. Basically, administrators are expected to enable realization of goals or desired future states by using information to plan programs or anticipate problems. Program managers also provide leadership by setting rules, inspiring workers, or developing objectives. In addition to performing these functions, managers also use information to gain and allocate resources, which help to renew the organizations they direct. Central to this function is the use of information to control the external environment.

Control of the environment may be too strong a phrase for a process of interorganizational negotiation. Furthermore, no organization has complete control over its environment, and organizations in the public sector are vulnerable to changes in state or federal policies. Perhaps it is more accurate to say that managers of public community service programs *attempt* to control the environment in which they function, protecting what they have built (e.g., in going after dollars, rather than directing and tracking services). Community service systems for the mentally retarded and developmentally disabled are in need of special management strategies, since some features of the external environment are now unpredictable. In addition, the growth of the privately operated residential care system, coupled with continued public responsibility for the welfare of clients, has created new adversaries.

Complicating the service effort is the limited community support for residential alternatives, such as group homes in suburban or city middle-class neighborhoods. Both public and voluntary agencies sometimes encounter resistance from neighbors. While no evidence exists that home values decline when residential programs of modest size are established near them, managerial energies are often excessively absorbed in efforts to overcome community resistance. Generally, managers make progress by establishing one small residence at a time in many different locations. It is interesting that low-income and working-class communities are more receptive than affluent communities to group homes and to family care. Independent living arrangements for retarded adults have been successfully installed in the social environment of rented apartments, particularly in declining urban areas where landlords have been cooperative in renting apartments for mentally retarded adults who have little need for direct services; yet parents are reluctant to see their vulnerable sons or daughters living in areas noted for higher than normal rates of violence.

Another problem is that a director of regional mental retardation programs cannot always maintain an adequate level of high-quality community services, because funding for nonresidential support services is most likely to be affected when cuts are imposed at the state level. For example, when "Proposition 13" imposed budget restrictions on regional centers in California, respite care for families was curtailed; concomitantly, admission rates to state hospitals jumped. Nonresidential services, including case management, home support and homemakers, in-person advocacy, counseling, family care, independent and supervised apartments, and habilitation, require personnel and space. When savings are sought, such community services are seen by state agencies as expendable. This results in state efforts to convert these personnel and other "line items" into federally reimbursable personnel lines and other than personnel expenses for ICF-MR facilities, with negative results on comprehensive community services. For example, two state-operated regional agencies in New York State with highly visible networks of storefront or community-based units, housing neighborhood-based service teams and specialized treatment programs, were forced to return to traditional care. Thus, low-cost but effective support services were substantially reduced in these communities as a result of the state's perceived need to recoup its investment in large developmental centers by filling the facilities with residents for whom reimbursement could be claimed at the much higher per diem allowed for care in an ICF-MR.

The experiences of these community service-oriented programs are not unique. Despite these difficulties, most managers of community service agencies believe that the goals and objectives of deinstitutionalization and the establishment of a continuum of community services are realizable. Stanley Nelson, a county service administrator from Lancaster County, Pennsylvania, has listed four goals and related objectives for his agency.

1. To promote the growth of persons toward higher levels of functioning, toward greater self-esteem, emotional maturity, competence and self-responsibility:
   • By influencing community systems (home, school, church, industry, government, health, human service, etc.) so that these systems become more affirming and growth-stimulating environments.
   • By facilitating the development of special growth experiences (i.e., education, training) for persons not identified as disabled.

- By facilitating the development of special growth experiences (i.e., coordinated treatment, habilitative, and rehabilitation services) for psychosocially and developmentally disabled persons.
2. To prevent the movement of persons toward lower levels of functioning:
   - By identifying high risk populations and facilitating the development of special experiences for such populations which enhance their personal skills.
   - By facilitating the development of programs which promptly intervene in and stop negative changes in people's functioning.
   - By influencing community systems which touch the lives of high risk and disabled persons so that those systems become more supportive and stabilizing environments.
   - By facilitating the development of specialized services which support and stabilize psychosocially and developmentally disabled persons who have reached their optimal growth.
3. To plan and implement an efficient program which effectively promotes growth and prevents disability.
4. To encourage and facilitate the participation of the citizens of the community in the attaining of these goals.

Managers of residential alternatives would agree with these goals, but would also insist that organizational problems make their attainment extremely unlikely. Of the more than 2,000 managers of community residential facilities surveyed in 1978, more than 85 percent mentioned staff turnover as a pressing problem. The second most frequently cited problem was funding.

Accountability

How does an agency like Lancaster Developmental Services demonstrate that it has achieved these goals and objectives? Agencies have to audit and review their programs to account for the expenditure of public and private funds and to demonstrate the effective and efficient use of their resources. Accountability drives the system. No longer considered an economical way to deal with the problem of mental retardation, community services for severely and profoundly retarded are costly (though usually less so than institutional care). As a result, its proponents are very careful to state the developmental argument for this type of service, emphasizing improved functioning and normal living.

Several issues of concern to managers of community service systems encourage the use of accountability techniques to assure responsible officials, parents, and the public that these programs are effective. Documentation is required on the procedures used to select clients and the benefits of community services. One major concern is whether seriously disabled clients can develop and change by use of this treatment modality, and whether the higher cost of delivery and the higher risk of clients' safety is worth the investment. Another concern has to do with the amount or sufficiency of community service. There are benefits for clients who remain with their families, and better home supports enable many clients to do so. Yet it is not clear how much in the way of home support is required; it has not been demonstrated that these benefits encourage independent or adaptive behavior. Similarly, we do not know the impact on the service system of family support programming. That is to say, is it possible to limit or reduce institutional beds through home support?

Professionals who administer community service systems are also concerned about the problem of maintaining quality control in a decentralized system, a configuration mixing public and private providers as well as different service models. Dispersed settings have a high potential for client abuse and neglect. Mental retardation professionals agree that quality assurance cannot be based solely on annual licensing visits or in-person case managers who drop in once a month. Citizens, neighbors, and parents who will act as advocates or personal representatives are also necessary to maintain humane standards. Quality assurance has been given new meaning by Lancaster County, which extends this concept to using citizen evaluators. A similar process is in place in Macomb and Oakland counties in Michigan. The need for monitoring dispersed care is central to the concept of community services. It would be tragic to reproduce one of the major flaws of large and isolated state schools by fostering a lack of accountability in more decentralized facilities.

Private vendors are increasingly used in various states to deliver residential services because they are quickly mobilized, economical, and efficient. It is easier for the states to deal with a few large vendors controlling "beds" in multiple locations than with many small providers. Large corporations, both profit and nonprofit, continue to enter the field, often faster than state agencies can develop adequate policies, standards, and monitoring mechanisms. The ever-expanding role of private sector care in the mental disabilities market, combined with changes in federal funding policies, could significantly reduce the accountability of service providers to the public.

Although the possibility exists that the private proprietary sector can provide humane and cost-effective care and services, its record is not extensive in the mental retardation field, although a few long-standing, well-known private nonprofit facilities have excellent reputations. Furthermore, most prior private sector management experience has been in the nursing home industry, a field which has seen many scandals. It is reasonable that many professionals are concerned and skeptical about the trend toward formation of vendor chains or cartels.

There are two ways to achieve accountability, i.e., to determine whether necessary services are delivered to the target population in an appropriate manner. The first technique is based on *outcome measures* of change in the behavior and/or attitudes of the target population. Such measures help to evaluate the impact of an innovation or a new service on the population served.

Outcome measures and controls are extremely difficult to establish and take a lot of time to perfect; nevertheless, they provide hard evidence that something works. To document that designated consequences follow from program designs, an outcome study may be employed to compare relative merits of the therapy versus another form of intervention. Controls are not likely to be built into such a design, as they might be in clinical drug trials, but some effort is made to limit random effects. Unlike theoretically relevant research, outcome studies do not try to explain how and why something works; they answer only the pragmatic question of *whether* it works and are used to evaluate programs such as probation alternatives to prison sentences as punishments, or income maintenance through a negative income tax.

The second technique of accountability is process-oriented. This type of design does not deal with the question of end results, but of whether the service is actually delivered. For example, it makes sure that speech therapy is provided for so many hours per week by an accredited therapist to a client in need of that service, or it measures the performance of the service unit in question according to the number of client contacts per month. Process measures are most effective when the techniques have already been proven to be beneficial to clients. These measures also need to be backed up by fiscal sanctions and incentives to ensure incremental service improvement. Therefore, graduated incentives and sanctions are essential components of any community living and habilitation oriented service accountability system.

The demand for information about the mentally retarded and the programs that serve them increases as those programs become more diverse and decentralized. Several forces contribute to this demand, ranging from professionals who plan and deliver services to individual clients, to those public officials who appropriate the funds for services at state and national levels. A common difficulty encountered by the state agencies in meeting these demands occurs when efforts are made to translate (present) existing information management systems in terms of contemporary information needs. "State of the art" studies have repeatedly suggested improvements in instrumentation and procedures requisite to the design and operation of management information systems to meet the emerging demands in the human service enterprise.

PROBLEMS IN ACCOUNTABILITY

A number of factors have hindered an even development of systems of accountability. One of the problems stems from the growth of the private sector in providing mental retardation and developmental disabilities services. Policy-makers who advocated rapid deinstitutionalization used purchase-of-service mechanisms, permitting public funds to be channeled to private sector caregivers. Early Medicaid policies made care for the mentally retarded, as well as psychiatric patients, reimbursible outside of state facilities.

In the 1970s several states decided to divest themselves of responsibility for direct care, depending instead on regional administrative units and local authorities to manage the burgeoning community-based system. Almost all these designated units were allowed to contract with a range of private agencies for the provision of residential and other community services. Some states, such as California, depended heavily on the use of board and care facilities not adequately governed by state certification and/or licensing provisions. Despite recent upgrading of certification standards, the capacity of localities to monitor such facilities is severely limited. New regulations for ICF-MRs, which provide fiscal support for active treatment, have stimulated even greater private sector growth in specialized residential services for the mentally retarded.

Various private sector providers have formed associations to aggregate and articulate their interests in state capitals and Washington. Inevitably, these associations have become additional voices in support of deinstitutionalization. Large corporate chains have entered the field of services for the mentally retarded. Thus, the community service system, through the mechanism of contracting out for services, has enhanced diversification, but also has increased the political power of the private voluntary agencies.

It is important to assess the implications of these changes for the new decade to make sure that this system is responsive to client needs. One significant change has been the involvement of large proprietary chains with multiple ICF-MRs or group homes in the same state or even in several states. The need for heavy capitalization makes it difficult for voluntary agencies and small proprietors to start residential programs. As control among a small group of large corporate entities increases, the power of the state and federal government to influence service directors and client priorities decreases. In some states with small populations, one or two providers can control a significant sector of the service system.

How are these providers monitored? Regional or county mental retardation services employ case managers, who are often responsible for staggering caseloads. In some states or localities, staff members specifically monitor or provide quality control. Yet local agencies, in many states, have little or no authority over licensing and certification of private mental disabilities agencies. Licensing and Medicaid certification may be vested in a generic agency, such as the state department of health, which is administratively separate from the mental health and/or mental retardation agency. Although some administrators of service systems for retarded persons may have some input into licensing and certification standards, many find themselves with little or no responsibility for on-site surveys and for the professional qualifications of staff empowered to survey and license these special purpose facilities.

In summary, there are several ways of enhancing public accountability in the provision of services to mentally retarded persons. At present, states should be alert to evaluate how much of the market can or should be controlled by one provider and to the possible long-term ramifications of allowing one corporate entity to develop a monopoly. Small providers should be encouraged; consumers must be offered a choice. The future demand for various types of facilities and services must be responsibly anticipated and planned. States should also stabilize those private sector residential programs considered desirable by maintaining adequate levels of reimbursement and developing contingency plans in the event of private sector discontinuation or poor performance.

Policy planners can avoid poor performance by developing a hierarchy of monitoring and quality assurance mechanisms at all levels of the system, paying particular attention to the client. Program content at private facilities would benefit by involving state, regional, and county mental retardation and developmental disabilities staffs in the preparation of licensing and certification standards, in surveying facilities, and in forging linkages of private residential facilities to the community service system.

Styles of Leadership

The goals of mental retardation services in the community are similar to those in many human service organizations—to induce clients to change. Agencies that provide regionalized community services for the mentally retarded must often resolve a variety of problems before change can be effected in the lives of clients. One central accomplishment has been the creation of residential alternatives to state schools, and where needed, to families when some kind of change in the life of the mentally retarded person is required.

Creating community services also makes feasible the deinstitutionalization of substantial numbers of mentally retarded persons who live at state schools or developmental centers. The formation of a family care program and an apartment living program was planned by one community-based agency, Bronx Developmental Services, as an alternative to large and isolated institutions. The formation of community service teams was designed to coordinate services for clients. Such services are now found both in specialized units created by this regionalized mental retardation agency and in more generic community-based facilities, such as the public schools in the case of educational services, or acute care hospitals for medical care. The community service teams helped to create services where none previously existed.

In attempting to develop community services in an urban setting, three units of Bronx Developmental Services were at the cutting edge of community programming. The Family Care Unit's goals were to find suitable caretakers in the community and to place and maintain mentally retarded of any age, including the severely retarded and multiply handicapped, in foster care. A second unit, the Northwest Bronx Community Services Team, one of the subregional interdisciplinary units concerned with a variety of services, had limited responsibility for providing residential care but was frequently concerned with the task of finding such residential care primarily in the form of care in the community. This program, it should be noted, dealt with families in extreme situations or crisis, who often appeared to be unable to manage a mentally retarded person any longer in the household. This problem frequently emerged in families with elderly and/or infirm parents. The third unit, the Independent Living Program, attempted to place mentally retarded adults in apartments with one or more roommates, most of whom, but not all, were also mentally retarded.

The authors' lengthy professional association with these programs affords a close look at the styles of leadership in these units. One might anticipate that the personalities of the unit managers might shape how they supervise and lead their subordinates or, alternatively, that managers would be attracted to their units according to vocational interests and personal experience. Regardless of how this happened, three distinct styles of leadership were fitted to the task at hand. These styles were located in the relationships established by supervisors with staff and shaped by the work experience and goals of the unit.

When perusing the subsequent elaboration of these styles of leadership, the reader should realize that certain limits are built into all human services agencies: (a) the members of most units have a variety of educational and vocational backgrounds; (b) the managers often have to act as advocates for their units and, therefore, spend a great deal of time competing with each other for resources; and (c) the norms of professionalism restrict close supervision or the use of punitive techniques for maintaining productivity and effectiveness.

As a further word of caution, it should be understood that the three distinct professional styles of unit management, designated as *rationality*, *control*, and *inspiration*, are ideal types and deliberately stress the differences between managers. Aside from their evident commitment to the clients of the agency, these managers all share the beliefs that effective case management makes community maintenance of the mentally retarded possible. Where they differ is in the level of involvement with clients and their families, the criteria used to evaluate case workers, and the importance of external resources for creating a successful change in clients.

To assess models of unit management one must determine, first, how they fit the task at hand, whether they can be extended to new tasks, and whether they are in accord with new philosophies and techniques in the human service field. Second, the emergence of these models may serve as a critique of current tendencies in human service management and practice. In particular, the current vogue for community care for the mentally retarded and developmentally disabled is based on notion that being in the community is a magic unto itself that will help clients. The nature of the clients involved in community care is considered almost irrelevant, and the degrees of disability, interchangeable. Yet it will be shown that quality of case management is a key element to successful community placement or maintenance of clients with families in the community. It can be used to facilitate just about any intervention; alternatively, if it is meant to be a more limited intervention, it would be insufficient as a technique for maintaining persons in the community. Finally, the role of the unit manager in community care needs some illumination, whether case management is strictly used or not.

PROFESSIONAL RATIONALITY: THE FAMILY CARE UNIT

Professional rationality may be defined as the use of established social work investigative techniques and the competent application of knowledge of child development theory (or a similar body of knowledge) to accomplish predictable and standardized tasks. The unit manager is able to delegate responsibility because many of the tasks are accomplished by following established, proven procedures. Moreover, in these cases the unit's goals are achieved by performing cumulative and interdependent procedures.

The most predictable features of the work of the Family Care Unit are the location of, training of, and certification of caretakers. In addition, the work includes the evaluation of clients prior to placement and the evaluation and support of caretakers once placement is made. Much careful investigation and selection of eligible caretakers precedes client placement. The unit manager employs a safety officer to make sure that domiciles comply with building codes, etc.; that new rules concerning fire extinguishers and smoke detectors, for example, are followed by caretakers; and that problems are cleared up, where possible, before placement is made.

Caretakers are selected on the basis of economic, social, and psychological criteria. Case workers determine whether a potential caretaker will be easy or difficult to supervise, and relations between case workers and caretakers are "cultivated" so that dependable caretakers will maintain their placements and consider accepting other placements. Most of the clients' problems are dealt with directly by the caretaker, with the guidance of the professional staff. But caretakers themselves can present difficult problems to the case worker. Thus supervision by the case worker sometimes involves classical psychotherapeutically oriented support and opportunity for caseworkers to vent feelings about a caretaker.

The unit manager is also concerned about retaining workers trained to perform the various tasks of the Family Care Unit. The maintenance of a stable staff with little turnover is a source of pride to the unit manager, because experienced and knowledgeable case workers are most important to the successful selection of caretakers and the placement of clients. Enthusiastic intervention in the lives of caretakers and clients may produce short-run gratifications for all but may eventually lead to "burn out" of staff and caretakers. The particularistic relationship established between case workers and caretaker is often intense, and transfer or termination of employment by a worker is upsetting to the latter. Caretakers may perceive such transitions as tantamount to abandonment by a trusted professional.

The unit manager was also concerned with the need to accord recognition to caretakers, to maintain their confidence in the agency, and to give them more timely compensation for hidden costs. The Family Care Unit of the Bronx Developmental Services regularly held a Parent Appreciation Day, raising money through team efforts. The staff also considered client participation in the Special Olympics, along with active participation in programs associated with the International Year of the Child. The unit manager also noted the need for more authority—that control over the budget for special purchases for clients or caretakers should be directly administered by her unit. Credibility with caretakers depended on being able to deliver on needed items, which also enhanced the unit's influence. Along these lines, the unit manager felt that reimbursement to caretakers for damages caused by clients to homes would be an important incentive in gaining access to new caretakers and keeping the old.

Professional rationality, in sum, is a model of supervision based on *predictable tasks* and the plausible assumptions that (a) planning will produce results and (b) emergencies will be relatively infrequent. Under those conditions the work of planning will *not* have to be suspended. Many of the predictable, but additional, tasks of the unit, such as planning summer camp placements, orienting or supervising new workers, etc., can be absorbed and assigned because scheduling can be maintained.

PROFESSIONAL CONTROL: THE NORTHWEST BRONX COMMUNITY SERVICES TEAM

Professional control may be defined as supervision of the techniques of advocacy and short-term intervention which, by definition, are limited involvements with the client and the family. The task specialization found under professional rationality did not occur here, except that case workers were encouraged to enrich their work and the unit itself by developing individual projects to serve many clients. Workers were expected to take on cases when the unit manager determined a match between client and worker. The members of the team were drawn from different disciplines; each worker's individual expertise was recognized as a resource when he or she became knowledgeable about such aspects of human services as community agencies, the welfare system, or the Office of Vocational Rehabilitation. Supervision was direct, and professional authority was not granted to each worker; the worker was not considered to be in the best position to judge what techniques to utilize or services to acquire.

Here is an example of how supervision works: The Northwest Bronx Community Service Team tends to come into contact with clients when they are in distress or when their families face cyclical crises. As a community service team that reaches clients *in extremis*, the temptation and opportunity to become deeply involved as a psychotherapeutic agent is very great. In staff meetings and in supervisory conferences with staff, the unit manager determines how therapeutically involved the case workers have become with clients and sets limits on the level of involvement. The unit manager stresses advocacy for the clients to help develop a trusting relationship in which clients, when possible, learn to advocate for themselves.

The type of supervision engaged in by the unit manager stresses productivity in the service of the client. Meeting deadlines, keeping up-to-date case records, and identifying unmet needs are competencies stressed to effect change in the client's life. In turn, the unit manager learns about the characteristics of the client and the need for new programs in case conferences and in supervisory sessions. Short-term therapy conducted by workers, with limited goals, is permitted; supervision is not psychother- apeutically oriented. Workers are trained to evaluate programs with which the unit manager may not be familiar, and are not expected to perform tasks available in other parts of the agency's network of services, e.g., psychologi- cal testing or therapy. By and large, the unit manager attempts to keep the workers working for the clients as advocates, and to bring individual projects into being. In this way, the style of professional control is equivalent to Peter Drucker's "Management by Objective."

When families are in crisis there are no easy predictions as to when that crisis will be resolved. Given the unpredictable character of the problem- solving required for clients and families in distress, and the indeterminate nature of the length of search for a solution, strong direction of the unit's resources is the most feasible way to organize a community service team. This raises questions about staffing. One might question whether staffs need persons with professional degrees, particularly those trained as psychiatric social workers, nurses, or psychologists. Moreover, staff members with experience in other agencies or units where they had more autonomy and were encouraged to become therapeutically involved with the client might have developed a "trained incapacity" for advocacy work. Therefore, selection of staff is extremely important for professional control to operate as a management model. At the same time, it is possible that responsible workers with little prior professional training could do the job.

Finally, professional control as a model of unit management is similar to professional rationality, insofar as resources are required to maintain the cooperation of clients and their families. Maintaining the credibility of clients, particularly where psychotherapeutic activities are limited by unit policy, may be needed to develop the staff's reputation to be able to deliver the services needed by clients when requested. Similarly, the availability of alternatives to institutional care or respite services can become critical resources for families in crises.

PROFESSIONAL INSPIRATION:
THE APARTMENT LIVING PROGRAM

Professional inspiration may be defined as the use of the *worker* as the major human resource to change the client. The occupational behavior most utilized is the personal involvement of the case worker in the life of the client. The worker is the role model for the client, as well as the benefactor, just as the unit manager is the role model for staff. The emphasis is on instruction and interpretation of the rules of society for the client, particularly for those socialized to live with their families or who previously lived in state schools.

Clearly, the idea of professional inspiration comes from that form of authority associated with being considered special, called *charisma* by

Weber. The possessor of charisma or extraordinary talent is often listened to because he or she occupies an office. Unit management by inspiration requires the constant presence of the manager to remind the staff of their mission. Unlike the manager who claims that people who take work home with them are wasting their working day, the professional inspiration manager views the job of the case worker as twenty-four hours a day. Staying late to do extra work is the ideal form of involvement with the role of the case worker.

The Apartment Living Program provided living quarters for mentally retarded adults in the community and arranged the implementation of support services for the client. A great deal of direct guidance was also provided by the case worker. Unlike Family Care and the Community Service Team, this unit, which provided direct residential care in the community for mentally retarded adults, was not assisted by natural families or caretakers: the case workers and homemakers are the "front line" staff.

The client population was not noted for their capacity to fully care for themselves; they frequently get in trouble; they were often difficult to locate when not in trouble. The Apartment Living Program tried to reduce the number of emergencies to which they must respond by instituting a weekly 45-minute consultation between case workers and clients. Yet it was not unusual for staff to be called away from scheduled meetings to find a lost client-resident or to mollify an irate landlord when clients were sloppy in their housekeeping.

The staff were encouraged to view themselves as making deep commitments to clients. The program itself was defined by the director as a lifetime commitment, and he himself works an 80-hour week. Rather than delegate responsibility or limit intervention, the unit manager encouraged involvement. Staff were often exhorted to "be the older brother and sister. Do the rites of initiation." Each case manager carried only a small case load, but the expectations were that every client was unique and unpredictable. Therefore "every relationship is a new relationship, and the worker has to be there charting new course." Consequently, knowledge and experience counted for much less than enthusiasm and a capacity to stick to the client. The greatest flaw was disengagement from work, which represented the failure of inspiration.

Workers were rarely selected according to professional degrees; instead the recruitment interview was designed to look for a "sense of excitement and initiative." The unit manager selected his staff according to his being inspired by them and their potential for what they can do within the unit and for which clients. With unpredictable clients, this may be a viable procedure. In sum, professional inspiration defined a relationship, rather than a set of tasks as to what is "achievable."

Leadership represents the hard-to-define quality that can spell the difference between a client-oriented attitude and one of bureaucratic indifference. The common themes in the success of the three leaders and their respective units, despite the difference in management style, is (a) concern about the welfare of the clients and their families; (b) an emphasis on a supportive relationship for families, direct care staff, or service staff with greatest responsibility for the client; (c) the visibility of the leader or unit director who, in his own unique way, responded, and responded promptly, to staff who sought him out; and (d) the establishment of an *esprit de corps* among their staff, who were made to feel that what they are doing is important and makes a difference for their clients.

Therefore, in viewing the success of an agency's community-based operation, it is apparent that community location in itself is not a panacea. Clients and their caretakers need to have support supervision and to have their rights protected even in an atmosphere of enthusiasm. It must be recognized that overprogramming can be inhuman and adverse in its effects, reducing the person to sheer clienthood. Leadership, at its best, is a self-correcting force in community services for people who cannot fully take care of themselves.

10

Funding Community Services in the 1980s

The tragedy of mental retardation in a family is often initially expressed in terms of emotional pain and anguish. The family must bear other costs as well. In our country, more so than in other industrialized societies, the burden of mental retardation is shouldered, first, by the family, assisted to some extent by voluntary associations and, second, by the state, municipal, county, and federal governments. In some instances, as in the case of education and vocational training, the ultimate economy in public dollars, resulting from independence, self-sufficiency, and/or decreased dependence on the part of disabled persons, is obvious. Many mentally retarded persons are self-supporting; other cases may need a lifetime of support and protective services, requiring personnel and physical space.

In 1979, national expenditures for mental retardation services were estimated at $10.7 billion, with an estimated $4.2 billion of that figure provided by the federal budget. An April 1984 report from the Department of Health and Human Services, Office of the Inspector General, estimated that the total 1983 federal and state expenditures for services to the developmentally disabled had become $14.33 billion ($6.93 billion federal), and the overall cost continues to increase.

There has been growing acceptance of the idea that society and the family both share responsibiity for caring for persons affected by mental retardation. Over the years the growth of the proportion of total expenditures paid for by the federal government has reflected this commitment. A recent analysis by William C. Copeland of the Hubert H. Humphrey School of Public Affairs indicates that more than 400,000 citizens receive public support to offset the cost of their residential care in state institutions for the mentally retarded or mentally ill. This figure includes clients receiving community care services in skilled nursing care facilities, ICF-MRs, and other residential programs. In addition, about 1.3 million persons receive some form of public income maintenance or service while living independently or with their families.

This trend toward social integration is part of a larger commitment. The beginning of the modern era of social welfare legislation in the United States is traced to the Great Depression of the 1930s. During that national emergency, all elements of American society agreed that personal survival, minimal income, protection of health, and provision of other human needs were more central to the purposes and goals of society than maintaining classical principles of property rights.

The Social Security Act of 1935 was designed to assure a minimum income for certain categories of dependent persons—the elderly, exceptional and other needy children, and the blind. Through subsequent amendments in 1950 and 1956, these provisions were extended to all types of disability that affect economic independence. A similar approach was advanced through federal grants-in-aid to states for vocational rehabilitation and for education for the handicapped. Current federal funding for community programs and to improve existing public institutions is dependent on the various entitlements created under amendments to the Social Security Act.

Entitlement programs are those for which legislation requires the payment of benefits to any person who, or government (on the state or local level) which, meets the requirements established by such a law. Entitlement programs are designed to have long-term and far-reaching effects. Until recently they were considered stable and reliable sources of funds, but many are now in jeopardy as a result of attempts to put ceilings on entitlement programs, to change eligibility criteria, and to place the entitlement programs and other funding sources in block grants. In addition, specific discretionary or project grant authorities have always been vulnerable to efforts to reduce expenditures in the health and social service parts of the federal budget.

Substantive changes in law are required to alter the entitlement programs, since the Executive Branch of the federal government cannot reduce expenditures for these items unilaterally. Steps have already begun both in the Executive Branch and in Congress to limit outlays through the entitlement mechanisms, and there is a definite trend to put ceilings on or cut back on social programs. This began with the enactment of a ceiling on Title XX (Social Services when it became law in 1975.) In 1980 Congress approved decreased Social Security benefits to families of disabled workers who became eligible for disability insurance.

Federal funding patterns, indirectly as well as directly, affect the availability of community services for the mentally retarded. Certain federal statutes foster services for this population, while new financial burdens are added to local and state governments through the requirement for matching federal dollars. Yet the appropriations to assure provision of the new service obligations are not always forthcoming from the federal budget. In the case of education for the handicapped, where receipt of federal dollars carried a much larger obligation, counties and municipalities are not necessarily able to assume the mandated costs. Moreover, local officials are often left to deal with the recriminations of angry and frustrated constituents, spurred on by rising expectations for services.

The major sources of federal support for the mentally retarded come from expenditures authorized under provisions of the Social Security Act. In 1977, approximately 83 percent of the Department of Health, Education and Welfare's financing of services for the mentally retarded came from these sources. By contrast, only 11 percent of the total departmental expenditures were through traditional federal formula grant-in-aid (state entitlement) programs, such as vocational rehabilitation, maternal and child health, aid to crippled children, and education of the handicapped and persons with developmental disablities.

Three actions taken by Congress in the 1960s and 1970s articulated a specific federal responsibility for the basic "safety net" for handicapped persons. In 1965 Congress enacted Title XIV, providing federal financial participation in state programs of medical assistance to the categorically needy, including adults with mental and physical disabilities. In 1974 it extended Medicare to disabled Social Security beneficiaries. Second, the Supplemental Security Income (SSI) Program enacted in 1972 guaranteed minimum federal cash assistance to needy aged, blind, and disabled persons (Title XVI). During fiscal year 1981, mentally retarded SSI recipients received federal benefits totaling more than $1.1 billion. By 1983, Social Security Income maintenance programs, including SSI and SSDI, totalled $2.3 billion. (In addition, many states also supplement SSI with additional payments to eligible people, with an estimated $580 million expended in 1983.) Third, federal aid became available in 1972 to cover the cost of intermediate care services as an optional Medicaid-reimbursable service (Title XIX). Federal-state outlays for ICF-MR services increased from $871 million in fiscal year 1977 to a total cost of $3.6 billion by 1983. The ICF-MR program is the most rapidly expanding source of federal support for the mentally retarded, and is becoming the states' major source of reinbursement for providing residential care. Finally, in the early seventies, with no specific federal targeting for mentally retarded and other developmentally disabled persons, a variety of protective and supportive services, including early intervention, day care, counseling, foster care, respite care, advocacy, and homemaker services, began to receive federal funding through state allocations under what later became Title XX (in 1975). As is the case in other federal programs, the states largely determine the specific services to be provided. Approximately $300 million dollars in federal funds, matched by another $100 million, is expended by the states for these services for mentally retarded persons. Title XX funding is an entitlement program for states on a shared allocation proportional to their population. The proportion of the total allocated for mental retardation services varies considerably from state to state. Other generic health and social services, partly paid for by the federal government and not included in these figures, also reach mentally retarded persons. Nonspecialized long-term care, acute hospital care, outpatient care, and generic social services also provide assistance to eligible individuals.

Federal assistance in other programs for the poor or disabled are important sources of community services, helping the recipient remain economically viable outside of 24-hour care. The Food Stamp Amendments of 1979 provide that disabled persons, who reside in public or nonprofit living arrangements that are properly certified and serve no more than sixteen residents, are eligible for food stamps. This amendment renders mentally retarded persons residing in group homes or hostels eligible for food stamps. Residents in these facilities are often also eligible for SSI, whether the facility is public or private. (SSI is not available in nonmedical public residential facilities serving more than sixteen people.) Additional assistance to community living has been provided by the Housing and Community Development Act of 1974 (Section Eight). This statute provides a means by which low-income families and elderly or handicapped individuals can afford decent housing. Eligible tenants in new or rehabilitated housing contribute no more than 25 percent of their gross income to rent, and the government subsidizes the landlord for the balance to the extent of a "fair" rental value, are determined for each location.

When the amendments recognizing the concept of "intermediate care facility services for the mentally retarded" (ICF-MR) were introduced into the federal legislative pipeline in 1970, authority already existed for federal participation in the cost of "intermediate care" for adult aged or disabled welfare recipients who required "institutional" care and were in private facilities offering more than board and lodging but less than skilled nursing care. Federal reimbursement for public assistance or care under Medicaid was available only to persons in a medical institution, and institutions for the retarded were not considered "medical" unless they qualified as hospitals or skilled nursing facilities. As a result, by 1970 some states had begun to convert their public facilities to nursing homes, and others began a massive exodus of residents who would be eligible for public assistance in community or private facilities, including but not limited to nursing homes, a process generally perceived as "dumping."

In passing the ICF-MR amendment late in 1971, Congress had three objectives in mind: (a) to give retarded persons in public facilities the same entitlements as those in private facilities; (b) to neutralize incentives to move retarded residents for fiscal gain without programmatic advantage to them; and (c) to offer assistance to the states in upgrading the quality of care and "active treatment" in what had become, for the most part, "custodial" settings. It was recognized that "public" did not have to equate with big and bad, and that private facilities were not necessarily all small, beautiful, and accountable. Nor did the legislation stipulate that only private facilities could qualify under the new clause [Section 1905 (d) of the Social Security Act]. As it turned out, states have chosen to apply the same standards to both, when the facility, whether public or private, assumes the round-the-clock, seven-days-a-week responsibility for both maintenance and program direction.

Meanwhile, President Nixon, at the suggestion of the President's Committee on Mental Retardation, had articulated the objective of returning one-third of the residents of public institutions to the community by 1980. This objective, briefly titled "deinstitutionalization," was taken seriously within the then Department of Health, Education, and Welfare, although responsibility for its attainment was somewhat diffuse. Concurrently with the enactment of the ICF-MR amendment and the adoption of "deinstitutionalization" as a presidential objective, the new Developmental Disabilities Services and Facilities Construction Act, signed by President Nixon in October 1970, began to take effect. Its National Council took an active part in interpreting the complexity of the "deinstitutionalization" movement as applied to persons considered retarded or developmentally disabled. A formal position was promulgated recognizing that there must be a least three components: (a) prevention of institutionalization by providing alternatives in the community; (b) discharge of residents already admitted on an individualized basis with adequate community support; and (c) "institutional reform." Institutional reform encompassed the two objectives of giving the institution the capacity to prepare residents for transition to the community and of providing a safe, humane, and habilitative environment for those who remained (for whatever period) in the institution. It has not been federal policy to consider persons already admitted to public institutions as expendable in any social experiment. These policies received "generic" reinforcement by the executive or legislative branches in the goal statements incorporated under Title II in Section 1904.

The foregoing was entirely consistent with the decision of Judge Frank Johnson, in the landmark case of *Wyatt* v. *Stickney* decided in 1972. His order, as it applied (and applies) to the Partlow State School and Hospital in Alabama, embodied all these principles. In addition, it enunciated explicit staffing standards and civil rights protections, including due process procedures and use of "least restriction" measures. All these were in hand as the federal government moved to promulgate regulations (standards) for implementation of the new Section 1905(d) of the Social Security Act. (The recent Supreme Court decision on the Pennhurst case may nullify some of these standards, however.)

In Section 1905, Congress used the term "active treatment." This meant that some criteria other than sponsorship (public, voluntary of proprietary) should be primary in determining the extent to which federal aid might be forthcoming. The criteria were intended to have something to do with quality, safety, and affirmative impact on the residents (habilitation). The Secretary of Health Education and Welfare (now Health and Human Services) was, therefore, mandated to set standards, provided that in matters of life and safety he took his cues from those standards already mandated for nursing homes.

Proposed standards became the subject of great effort—both by those within government responsible for quality control and by those consumer spokesmen, providers, and state agencies who would be heavily impacted. The standards developed by the Accreditation Council on Facilities for the Mentally Retarded became the basis for proposed federal standards. Within the federal establishment a basic conflict became apparent, in which the issue of probable impact on the federal budget became a central theme. Should standards be set high so that few facilities (states) could or would seek to comply with them, or should they be set low so that per capita cost could be contained at modest levels, even though more facilities would qualify? In the end, the proponents of "high standards" prevailed.

The high standards dealt with "active treatment," staffing requirements, and the like; they also applied to physical plant so that fire safety and plumbing became compliance issues. Compliance issues involved retro-fitting facilities already in existence, an action that became a prerequisite for future funding. The most costly and controversial parts of the "physical" mandates, however, related to the rooming standards. These were based on existing standards for skilled nursing facilities of not more than four beds to a room and a stated number of square feet for each bed. (It is curious that little attention was given to other kinds of space requirements for people who typically did not spend much time in their bedrooms.) Converting dormitories for sixty persons into fifteen bedrooms for four each became a major capital investment issue. Given the existing plants, populations would have to be reduced, and this requirement has in fact added considerable impetus to the push for depopulation. No state, whether in or out of the ICF-MR program, expected to increase the capacity of most of its public facilities; however, some found renovation of existing facilities less cost-effective than replacing them with new smaller, "more homelike" units built to new standards, but on the same grounds or in the community. State borrowing to finance such capital costs became manageable in view of the fact that the costs of interest and amortization can be built into the per diem attributed to future occupants, and hence shared with the federal government, as long as ICF-MR services remain optional under open-ended state and individual Medicaid entitlements.

A study by the National Association of State Mental Retardation Program Directors has revealed that, in the triennium 1977-79, states committed close to one billion dollars to pay for renovation and replacement of buildings in public institutions. These commitments occurred in states with and without ICF-MR programs; however, many state directors made it clear that they were motivated by the pressure to come into compliance with the ICF-MR standards by 1982. Considering that the current operating costs of public facilities now far exceed $1 billion a year, this investment in physical plant, large as it is, does not seem excessive. What worries many proponents of community care is the effect that this investment has or will have on future plans for further phase-down (or phase-out) of the larger public facilities. States will clearly be reluctant to abandon nearly new or expensively renovated buildings on which there is still a mortgage, represented by outstanding state bonds.

There is an important distinction between the requirement to reduce overcrowding (represented by the minimum floor area per bed) and the requirement to repartition or replace dormitories so that no more than four persons will sleep in one room. The former is a force for depopulation without additional investment; the latter is a force for major capital investment and tends to stabilize the institutional population at the level found at the specified compliance date.

During the 1977–79 triennium, state MR agencies also reported investing $98,091,000 in purchase or construction of community residences directly or through grants-in-aid or loans to voluntary agencies. In addition, housing for various day services was supported to the tune of $73,810,000. In comparing these figures with the much greater investment in reconstruction at the larger facility sites, it is important to recognize that capital funds for community construction are coming not only from state MR agencies, but from private investors, private endowments, and from HUD financing in substantital amounts not included in the above totals. Nevertheless, diversion of more capital from existing facilities to newer, smaller, more localized units appears to be urgently needed.

The place of the "small" community-based ICF-MRs in the spectrum of residential services is much debated. The issue is confused when the term "ICF-MR" is applied loosely to group residences not certified as ICF providers. Contrary to opinion in some quarters, ICF-MRs are not primarily mechanisms for funding; they are service delivery models, derived from the characteristics of persons who, in the language of Congress, "because of their mental and/or physical condition require care and services (above the level of room and board) which can be made available to them only through institutional facilities." The model requires the operator of the facility to be responsible for meeting the needs of residents. The funding mechanism reflects this model. It takes the form of a vendor payment not controlled by the resident, his advocate, or his personal representative, and is intended to pay for board, lodging, and any needed service to which the resident does not have an independent entitlement under such state or federal legislation as the Education for All Handicapped Children Act or the Rehabilitation Act. To the extent that the resident has income from earnings, Social Security, savings account, or other sources, he may be required to contribute everything above $25 a month for a "personal needs allowance" to the vendor or to reimburse the state (and indirectly the federal government) for its outlays.

For providers, the attraction of such a reliable "all-in-one" payment is obvious. For consumers it often means access to "interstitial" services for which a noninstitutional payment mechanism is not available. Medicaid, in some states, will pay for certain services when provided in or through the ICF or SNF, which it will not cover under federal regulations or state plan options or both when provided to a person in his or her own home or other noninstitutional setting. Moreover, some consumers, especially those entitled to Social Security benefits that exceed the alternative SSI payments, may be eligible for care and maintenance when in an ICF-MR for which they would not be eligible under another funding mechanism.

These discriminatory provisions affect the mentally retarded and the chronically mentally ill, the frail elderly, and certain younger persons with massive physical handicaps. Considerable attention has been given within the Department of Health and Human Services and in congressional committees to a general need for facilitating services to such vulnerable people in noninstitutional settings, including senior citizen housing projects, various group quarters, and private homes. The special needs of mentally retarded children and adults are now being taken into consideration as policies in these areas are modified with the creation of waivers on a case-by-case basis to permit individuals to receive Title XIX reimbursement services outside traditional hospital or institutional settings. Such approaches need to be standardized and more widely applied to broader population groups of disabled citizens.

Community Funding Approaches

Further capital expenditures to implement present ICF-MR physical standards may benefit those mentally retarded persons who will remain in state schools, but they should not prevent further deinstitutionalization or the accelerated development of community care services. Several funding mechanisms are already in place on the federal and state levels that can, through change in regulation or interpretation of existing statutes, provide the necessary stable financial support for community services.

The success of the community care approach to service depends in considerable measure on federal funding, which in turn depends on a clearly defined social policy by the various government agencies, especially the Health Care Finance Administration. Such a policy should recognize community care as a priority. Part of this policy should foster further phasing down of institutional capacities at a rate commensurate with realistic goals for "quality" placements of former residents in individually appropriate community settings. Improvements at state schools or developmental centers must be focused on those services that clearly affect client health, safety, and preparation for transition. Incentives should be offered to states to encourage community placement for those institutionalized residents who could benefit from being in a less restrictive environment. Alternative community residential placement of clients would be easier if the states were permitted to continue to draw down the same federal reimbursement for a former ICF-MR institutional resident for at least a year after his transfer to the community, regardless of the type of appropriate setting and constellation of services offered. This would make the exceptional costs of transition less burdensome to the states. A similar inducement was offered in the past with respect to the federal subsidy for children in state-operated schools when these children rejoined their local school systems.

A community service approach to funding also depends on a public commitment by local and state agencies to foster the development of nontraditional services. While there is no proven magic number, professionals have found that smaller group homes, including ICF-MRs of from three- to fifteen-bed units, can provide residential care at reasonable rates. Nevertheless, it would be desirable to provide rehabilitative day activities in separate outside facilities directly funded by state agencies. The Health Care Financing Administration has not yet seen its way to encourage funding these services under Title XIX, and they are not widely available.

Expanded respite care, funded under Title XIX or XX, could also be made available to both the natural and foster families as part of a total constellation of needed community services. Flexibility in financing the care of the handicapped is now expanded under waiver provisions and options for Title XIX, making it possible for this service and some others to be offered to families, as stipulated in P.L. 97-35 and P.L. 98-248.

One- or two-hundred well-run community residences, with available coordinated support and protective services either in or away from the facility, are now preferred by professionals to one large isolated institution. If a small facility wishes to qualify as an ICF-MR, it must demonstrate that there is an active treatment plan for each client, containing individualized goals and a set of objectives for attaining them. Further, even when clients receive outside day activities, the objectives of the treatment plan must be achieved across settings, and the ultimate responsibility for this rests with the sponsor.

A major problem for community residential care not using this delivery model has been to locate funding for day center activities for mentally retarded persons deemed unsuitable for vocational rehabilitation and sheltered workshop placement. It is sometimes possible to subsidize these programs through medically prescribed "health-related" services, paid for under Medicaid reimbursement procedures. After the completion of a physical, psychological, and cognitive assessment, professional services recommended by the physician can be augmented. Individuals so entitled can then have a fully rounded treatment program, with federal and state funding components. Nonetheless, federal policy in this area has been ambivalent and even capricious. Some advocates are fearful that if Title XIX funding is relied upon as a primary support for adult day programming, the heavy medical orientation will shift the emphasis away from "developmental" programming. Application of the same concepts of "habilitation" and "active treatment" (accepted and funded in an ICF-MR facility) to the "ambulatory" care model of community day care would largely resolve this problem.

The Alternatives to the ICF-MRs

Bearing in mind the fiscal, statutory, and ideological constraints of the ICF-MR program, Copeland and Iverson (1980a) have offered the following model of semi-independent living, with a staff of six on-site personnel serving twenty-four residents. The staff should be defined as providing "health-related services" under the state Medicaid plan.

> Eight two-bedroom apartments, in a large apartment complex, would be rented to persons who have reached the level of independence which allows them to go out each day to a job, a sheltered workshop or a vocational training activity in a Developmental Achievement Center. There would be three persons per apartment ($140 per person rent per month). Each person would be eligible for the food stamp minimum ($10 per month). All persons would be

Table 10.1   Costs and Sources of Support for Apartments (in dollars)

Cost item	Title XIX	SSI	HUD Section 8	Food Stamps	State	Total
Staff	51,150				41,850	93,000
Rent		17,266	23,060			41,326
Food and other		51,780		1,440		53,220
Total costs	$51,150	$69,046	$23,060	$1,440	$41,850	$186,540

eligible for Section 8 rental subsidy. (Within Fair Market Rent maxima, HUD will pay all rent over 25 percent of client income.) Six staff would be available for assistance and supervision, paid an average of $15,500 per year (funded under Title XIX, at 55 percent Federal, 45 State).

For such a budget, the state matching would be about 22 percent (35 percent if no Section 8 support were available), a level that most legislatures would find acceptable. At the same time, the total cost would remain reasonable—under $8,000 per year for the residential services. (Workshop services, adult day programs, transportation, social services, and medical services would for some classes of residential clients add about $4,000 to $6,000 to the total package, most of which could be funded by Title XIX, Title XX, VR, or by state and local funds.

The Role of State Government

At a federal level there are indications of an intent to give block grants to states, thereby placing state governments in the position to use funds to respond to needs as they perceive them. Nevertheless, states are under considerable financial pressure to reduce service and at the same time be politically responsive to interest groups.

Although the large block grant that would consolidate many federal entitlement programs would both simplify procedures at a federal level and give the state more autonomy and flexibility, it has several serious side effects and negative consequences. In some recent instances it intensified rivalries for services between competing groups at state and local levels and resulted in even more bitter competition than if the total dollar pool were decreased.

One way of dealing with the problem within the state is to look for cost-effective programming. The purchase of care from large private ICF-MRs begins to look very appealing to state government because staff costs are low, owing to less unionization, fewer educational requirements for personnel not protected by a civil service system, and sharper management practices nurtured by the marketplace. Private entrepreneurs also can often come "on line" more rapidly than state agencies with a new facility. Some of these initial advantages of the private vendors may disappear with time, as workers unionize or higher standards of performance are demanded by accrediting bodies. State responsibility for community services for the mentally retarded and the developmentally disabled will undoubtedly remain, particularly since private providers shun or exclude the most severely disabled, those with multiple handicaps or acting out-clients.

State budget analysts still need to be convinced that reasonable community services are important for both humanitarian and fiscal reasons. Documentation must be provided that demonstrates that decent programming will produce better utilization of state and federal funds.

Finally, to preserve and expand community services in the face of austerity, timely budget information and good evidence of program effectiveness must be available. It would be far better for clients if program managers developed their own rational and accountable methods of designing and evaluating programs than to leave these tasks to fiscal managers who have an inadequate understanding of who the mentally retarded are and what they can be with appropriate treatment services in a more normalized but stimulating environment.

Part Three

Research and Evaluation

11

Research on Community Services

The 1970s saw the development of several viable and comprehensive community services systems for the mentally retarded. Investigations concerning the impact of such programs are starting to provide evidence that there are real benefits for clients, that failure rates are modest, and that the social environment does make a difference. The catchy slogans "least restrictive environment," "as close to normal as possible," and "maximum feasible participation" are translatable into programs that work, provided these principles are applied in the light of an even more important one: individualization.

Until as recently as 1975 there had been few studies on the utilization of residential alternatives for mentally retarded adults, adolescents, or children. The efforts to create effective halfway houses, hostels, group homes, and family care arrangements under current assumptions are very recent. The few prospective or followup studies that were carried out forty or fifty years ago did not make comparisons among different community residential alternatives or, if comparisons were made, focused mainly on criteria that we would consider less valid today. Consequently, policy formation in the area of residential services and deinstitutionalization suffered from a lack of information concerning the kind of community-based facilities that improve the quality of life and enhance the adaptation of the particular persons who may come under the label "mentally retarded."

Research on community services is particularly important today to validate public policy. The movement to deinstitutionalize and relocate mentally retarded persons to their home communities has not been approved by all professionals and parents, or for that matter by city fathers or homeowners. Some planners in state capitals are skeptical about the idea of returning large numbers of state school residents to communities that exhibit signs of economic and social disorganization. Deinstitutionalization and the development of comprehensive community-based services is a prioriy some perceive to be inconsistent with other desired ends, such as improving physical conditions or installing active treatment programs at traditional state institutions.

Some opponents of increasing the rate of transfers from state institutions to community arrangements have pointed to the glaring failures of deinstitutionalization and, in particular, to the misfortunes befalling many chronically mentally ill persons discharged from mental hospitals during the 1960s. They have criticized the actions undertaken in many states to move individuals into group homes, nursing homes, private and proprietary facilities, and even family care, some of which have admittedly resulted in poor care and inadequate supportive services. In some states, the argument continues, increased placement in the community and the closing of admissions to traditional institutions has led to an overloading of the service delivery system in the community. Impressions of this kind continue to be communicated, even when there are data to suggest that we do know what to do, how to do it, and for whom.

A number of basic questions on research on community services will be addressed in this chapter.

- What characteristics of what kinds of various residential facilities and living arrangements promote improved adaptive behavior, including care of oneself, social skills, and the possibility of independent living, and for what types of clients?
- Do residential alternatives and other community supportive services improve the quality of life, increasing extensive social interaction and greater individual choice in friendship, and are these improvements accompanied by less personal, social, and economic dependence on others?
- What characteristics of residential services in the community encourage adaptive behavior and improve the quality of life?
- What characteristics of clients correlate with ease of community adjustment, and what characteristics call for remedial interventions?
- To what extent are residential and other community services able to train clients for independent living through planned programming?
- Can we quantify suitable goals for "all deliberate speed" in developing the resources to welcome persons returned from the isolation of the institution?
- Is there a set of reproducible and transmittable techniques that constitute ways of making life in community residential alternatives as close to normal as feasible, and how close is really desirable, and for whom?

Research by sociologists, social psychologists, and psychologists has identified certain characteristics of residential environments that are significantly related to the level of adaptive functioning of persons living there. Hull and Thompson measured the impact of several individual, residential, and community variables on adaptive functioning of mentally retarded persons. Individual characteristics such as IQ accounted for some of the differences in adaptation. But environmental variables, such as access to outside vocational, educational and recreational activities, promotion of independence by staff, appropriateness of activities of daily living to community standards, and urban location, were far more important in explaining the differences among residents in adaptive behavior. Thus, persons with the same level of intelligence demonstrated greater or lesser self-care, depending on the characteristics of the residential facility. An important predictor of adaptive behavior was the extent to which resident independence was fostered through a regimen that included a variety of self-help and domestic tasks.

One important aspect of community residential living involves satisfying and productive interpersonal relationships. A number of studies have reported that mildly and moderately retarded persons who have not developed social skills also have very few friends in the community or at work. Without those skills, one may wonder how such mentally retarded persons get along in community-based residential alternatives. Several studies of group homes and their resident populations suggest that most mentally retarded persons can achieve lives that are closer to normal living than was previously thought possible.

Landesman-Dwyer and her colleagues observed the social behavior of mentally retarded residents in group homes. The informal group behavior, affiliations, and intense social relationships (friendships) were categorized. Moderately and mildly retarded persons were more oriented to others when in groups than were severely and profoundly retarded residents. The latter group did demonstrate social behavior, but the higher-intelligence group also displayed more appropriate switching from social to neutral behavior (and back again), according to whether they were in or out of the presence of peers and staff.

Residents were observed engaging in social behavior that involved cooperation in a division of labor (e.g., games or learning situations), in verbal and gestural communication. These forms of affiliative behavior were not as related to personal characteristics, such as sex or intelligence, as they were to (a) the size of the group home, (b) average intelligence of the residents of the home, (c) the sex ratio of the home, and (d) homogeneity of the residents' backgrounds, such as whether they were relocated from the same traditional institution.

Although residents in larger group homes affiliated or had social interaction more frequently than in smaller ones, a finding independently established in other studies, intense relationships were as likely to be found in both types of homes. Most social behavior occurred among pairs or in dyadic situations. "Friendships" were measured by a proxy-variable. Pairs were considered friendly if they spent more than 10 percent of the observed time periods together. Although residents appeared to affiliate with peers of similar intelligence, this relationship could be attributed to the fact that residents tend to be segregated by intelligence and, therefore, were more likely to affiliate with others of a similar level of functioning.

Adults who live in group homes of other residential alternatives often attend sheltered workshops, which provide further opportunity for social interaction and friendship. Berkson and Romer studied the social ecology of four sheltered workshops and a new residence. Again, differences in settings largely accounted for predicted variation in affiliation, independent of personal characteristics. Although older and mentally ill clients affiliated less extensively, neither degree of retardation, length of previous institutionalization, use of medication, nor presence of physical disabilities appeared to affect affiliation, independent of other variables.

Affiliation was measured by clients' preferences as well as their actual behavior. A program with no possible social choices would surely be viewed as highly restricting by retarded and nonretarded persons alike. Berkson and Romer also sought to find out what cognitive and physical characteristics were used in client selections of others as the basis for interaction. Since observations were limited, staff judgments were also incorporated in this study to increase the data available. Social choice estimates were not, however, very consistent across staff and client observations. There is clearly a need for more extensive and sophisticated research in this promising area.

Successful group home living is evidence that community residential services are effective. Furthermore, group home living is only one residential alternative and can be considered as a first step toward even more normal living. Experience in a residential facility can be viewed as maximizing independence within that setting or as preparatory for further independence.

In a two-year national followup study of 1,800 previously institutionalized clients, Bruinincks and associates found that less than one-fourth of the residents of group homes left in that period. Among those clients who left, more than 30 percent were living independently in the community; almost 18 percent were living in the home of a relative; and 6 percent were in family care placements. Less successful were those (over 10 percent) who were returned to traditional institutions, or the small number (less than l percent) who fell into the custody of the law; in addition, more than 25 percent were living in another community residential facility. Perhaps the most significant finding was that most of the clients were still residing in group homes after two years. Thus, the return rates reported in this national study were relatively modest. As will be discussed later, a more-recent body of literature identifies client behavior problems and poor social adaptations as the principle causes of client failures to adjust to life in community residences.

Critics of traditional institutions have condemned these organizations as overly protective, depersonalizing, and socially isolating. Size has often been considered the basis of these characteristics. While there are many reasons for favoring smaller facilities, the variable of size per se appears to be less important than other factors, including age of facility, turnover in staff, or training and motivation of staff.

Variables often confounded with size may explain the lack of a relationship, as observed in many studies, between the quality of the environment and the number of residents in a community facility. In comparisons of social environments between seven community residences and large traditional institutions using the same scale, scores were generally superior in the group homes.

In a study by Pratt and Luszcz, five areas were assessed: daily management practices, the physical environment, resident-community involvement, staff-to-resident communication, and staff attitudes. It is interesting that these dimensions of residential environment varied independently of one another, clearly indicating the continued need for highly differentiated evaluation techniques.

Poor physical arrangements are often found in large and isolated traditional institutions. That a physical environment is important should not lead to the inference that social relationships invariably result from a satisfactory ambiance. Physical structure sets limits to activities, but does not limit social invention. A facility may be beautiful and thoughtfully designed, but management practices may discourage client stimulation. Thoughtful management must include such measures as using community-based supportive services, enhancing staff-resident contact, and avoiding rules that impose block treatment on residents.

Oral communication is one area in which the physical environment, number of residents in a particular room, and staff practices interact. Large rooms containing many people disadvantage residents with intellectual or hearing impairments, especially in understanding directions or developing speech. Incidentally, this is a strong argument for increased use of nonverbal communications methods.

Although size per se does not normalize services, size makes such normalization possible. The literature on residential care for disabled children points to the importance of appropriate social organization and orientation to clients as the basis of teaching self-care and communications skills. Differences in organization or in staff orientation, which correlate with size, may be artifacts of the changing temper of the times. Client-oriented practices are more likely to be found in small, community residential facilities, which are often newer than large facilities. Frequently, the staff of new group homes is made up of energetic, committed, and well-educated, young, human service providers. Whether for children or adults, the close proximity of smaller facilities to the community also provides models that can foster independence. Finally, small-unit organizations can generate greater client-staff contact by limiting staff-to-staff contacts. With less opportunity to talk to other staff members, staff can spend more time conversing with and teaching clients. The question of who lives in a facility may be more important than the question of how many. An interesting finding in the importance of heterogeneous grouping is found in the social ecological studies of group homes and sheltered workshops. In one such study of social interaction, Berkson and Romer (1980b) found that the "average intelligence of peers was important in determining how affiliative individuals will be in a setting." The investigators (1980c) also suggest that settings in which less-intelligent clients are segregated from others may decrease their social interaction. "The presence of clients of relatively moderate intelligence is crucial to the social integration of a setting, since they are most likely to form relationships with clients of both higher and lower intelligence." The characteristics of the providers also seem important

to adequate adaptation to community living, whatever the global characteristics of the clients served at a particular facility. In a comparison of the
characteristics of family care homes, Suttes found that the one-fifth who
returned clients to state schools had less experience as caretakers than the
contrast group. Furthermore, family arrangements were significantly
related to these failures in community placement. Those providers who
returned clients to the agency had more relatives living at home but fewer
relatives living nearby than successful family care providers.

Given the characteristics associated with clients who were not maintained
in the community (to be discussed presently), these findings on family care
providers are not surprising. Surveys of managers of group homes did not
pinpoint the maladaptive behavior of clients as one of their major problems
in administration. Yet behavior problems *were* cited in 70 percent of the
cases wherein group home managers returned clients to traditional institutions. Furthermore, in a comparison of successful and unsuccessful
placements in family care for mentally retarded persons in Hawaii,
maladaptive behavior was strongly associated with the return of clients to
traditional institutions. Males were also more likely to be returned than
females.

It is possible that recidivism rates are low because providers do not wish to
lose reimbursement while waiting for a replacement for a client returned to a
traditional institution. We would expect, then, that a great deal of
maladaptive behavior would be tolerated. In one study, a random selection
of twenty group homes in the state of Washington were subject to close
observation of staff and residents. The resident subjects ranged from 9 to 68
years old, with 75 percent of the residents in the 16-to-36 year-old range. At
least 77 percent of the residents had previously lived in a state institution for
the mentally retarded. According to medical records, 10 percent of the
residents were classified as borderline, 28 percent as mildly retarded, 41
percent as moderately retarded, and 20 percent as severely and profoundly
retarded. Fifty-five percent of the residents observed were males, 45 percent
females.

Residents in institutions are often characterized as displaying many
bizarre, destructive, or stereotypical behaviors. In contrast, residents in
these group homes showed remarkably little undesirable, abnormal, or
stereotypical behaviors. The major influence on the occurrence of these
undesirable behaviors appeared to be the level of retardation. Individuals
who were classified as severely or profoundly retarded behaved in undesirable ways ten times as often as did individuals labeled mildly or moderately
retarded.

Social integration is a variable that may be used to represent satisfactory
adjustment to community placement. Extensiveness and intensiveness of
interaction or affiliation was largely accounted for by two personal
characteristics in the research by Berkson and Romer. While physical
attractiveness and desire for sociability were strong characteristics, it is not
clear in what way these traits affected affiliation. It is possible that the less
attractive could either be rejected by others or that they simply avoided

interaction. In any case, it should be noted that attractiveness was not linked to the lack of physical disability, but was an independent dimension of the person, having more to do with cosmetic qualities, clothing, and general demeanor. Indeed, one study focused on "before and after" acceptability of the same young adults who were specifically trained in grooming and social behaviors.

Some evidence, based only on training programs, suggests that it is possible to teach adaptive and social skills to clients as preparation for community living. Birenbaum and Seiffer have observed, in connection with the study of one of the very first efforts of resettlement, that former state school patients were not used to being among strangers and would often stare at them. In a vocational and residential demonstration project, mentally retarded adults were placed during a two-year period after participating in either an independent living program or a competitive employment training program. Clients were evaluated as to placement success in their respective situations (residence or job); 13 percent returned to one or the other training program. Successful placement in independent living was related to intelligence and demonstrated skills in symbolic operations, personal maintenance, clothing care and use, socially appropriate behavior, and functioning so as to employ academic skills. Successful employment was related to sensorimotor functions, visual-auditory processing, language, and symbolic operations skills. The major reasons for returning from a job to the competitive employment training program were inappropriate behavior and the need for more training. Returning from a community living placement was related to failure in activities of daily living skills, such as management of money, cleanliness of the apartment, social behavior, and preparation of meals.

When clients worked and lived in the community, success in employment was not related to success in independent living, a finding that has also been established by other investigators. What is significant by and large is that training programs do increase the adaptive behavior of most clients. Thus, it appears that these kinds of targeted training, if reproducible nationally, could help to reduce recidivism after deinstitutionalization and could lower the demand for support services in the community.

One constant concern has been the possibility that deinstitutionalization will overload existing community services. A New York State study assessed the impact of relocation efforts upon a community-based service system in one county. Changes in the characteristics of clients seeking services, the type of services they needed, and the nature of interagency relations were explored. The results of the study indicated that not only are more formerly institutionalized persons seeking services, but the needs of this population are different and more intensive when compared to other community clientele. These kinds of findings are to be expected as more and more multiply handicapped and severely retarded persons are relocated in community settings. Nevertheless, others have pointed out that many severely and profoundly retarded people still have never been institutionalized. Closeted at home, their socially regressed behavior requires the same intervention as for any formerly institutionalized individual. Many of these individuals may still not receive services. It is somewhat difficult to assess whether community services are being overloaded to the point where clients suffer extreme neglect. A recent survey of superintendents of traditional state institutions supports the view that their surrounding catchment areas are facing difficulties as a result of deinstitutionalization. Furthermore, the need for greater access to supportive services is a continual complaint of parents of retarded persons living in the community. Indeed, recurring evidence shows competition for services and funding between the families of clients who were never institutionalized and always lived in the community, and the families of those returned as a result of deinstitutionalization.

Implications

A number of important implications of this recent research on community services should be addressed both by those who operate residential programs and by policy-makers. First, environments that encourage the acquisition of adaptive skills enhance the quality of life by fostering appropriate staff behaviors, allowing them to focus on interactions with clients in a way that encourages independence. Residential facilities can be planned so that the mix of clients sustains social interaction and friendships. Friendships are important to some mentally retarded persons, and they should be taken into account when shifts from one facility to another, whether residence or workshop, are considered. Second, adaptive skills can be taught. The technology of normalization appears to be available and can be transmitted to staff. It is possible to introduce "normalization," in its various forms, in many kinds of units. Third, clients can learn to appreciate the company of their peers and make more of an effort to seek them out. Similarly, their attractiveness can be increased through appropriate dress, cosmetics, and demeanor, all aspects of the self that can be altered. Future research should be directed to a focus on the verification of these findings.

12

The Managed Community

Introduction

Many retarded persons, mainly adults, are now living in community residences, group homes, family care homes, or independent apartments. These living arrangements represent a dramatic change in policy, following the Scandinavian principles of normalization and deinstitutionalization developed during the 1960s. The aim of this policy was to create coordinated but uncentralized programs in the community, making living conditions for mentally retarded persons as close as possible to the mainstream of society.

A number of mental retardation agencies incorporated these principles of normalization and deinstitutionalization into their models of highly accountable, state-run services. During a three-year period, Bronx Developmental Services, a regional branch of New York State's Office of Mental Retardation and Developmental Disabilities, received funds from the Office of Human Development, U.S. Department of Human Servces, for a demonstration project. This project attempted to create a single class system of care for the mentally retarded and developmentally disabled to correct the traditional, unsatisfactory, dual approach of providing segregated institutional care on the one hand, and limited, fragmented community-based services on the other.

Included in this project of national significance was the study of clients and their families, the effects of community-based residential services, and new forms of organizing domicilary care. These projects were among the first to report on community living, providing evidence of various kinds on the consequences of establishing community residential programs.

Since the middle of the last decade the number of mentally retarded persons living in various community settings has increased enormously. As reported in 1983, 57,494 persons, including 85 percent over the age of eighteen, reside in more than 6,300 group homes of various sizes and types. In addition, thousands of mentally retarded adults live in independent apartment units without daily supervision and thousands more in family care homes.

The case study that follows, and Chapters 13 and 14, examine the social environments in the different types of programs providing residential services, and the ways in which mentally retarded adults serve to influence this environment. These case studies help us to consider the following questions.

- What happens to mentally retarded adults, particularly those persons relocated from large and isolated state schools, when they live in a community residence?
- Do the high-functioning mentally retarded adults in independent apartment living programs develop patterns of mutual aide with those who are similarly situated and with their neighbors?
- What stressful impact does family home care have on the caretakers, and how do they cope with the strains that may occur?

In addition, these case studies can provide direct information within the local community agency to supplement or validate the data collected by a management information system. Participant observation and field interviews offer a different perspective on what is going on; practitioners in intake interviews and ongoing contact with the client may not be aware of the range of problems and accomplishments in the case of each client. In this way, social science research methods within the agency serve to monitor the quality of programs, providing periodic feedback to practitioners about their efforts that will help guide service delivery and allocate scarce resources.

A longitudinal-study approach to deinstitutionalization is useful as a means of evaluating policies and theoretical import, insofar as it makes possible the testing of concepts about the impact of social environments on the behavior, attitudes, and social relationships of mentally retarded individuals. Similarly, a longitudinal case-study approach to deinstitutionalization makes it possible to determine whether new residential programs in the community are able to maintain changes in behavior, attitudes, and social relationships initially manifest when residents of large and isolated state schools are returned to the communities where they once lived. The social ecology of the larger community in which residences are located may encourage or discourage greater or lesser levels of social and recreational participation. Even changes in lifestyle brought about by involvement in vocational rehabilitation programs may have some impact on available time and energy for using resources in the wider community. Being part of a social unit linked to a residence but with free access to diverse vocational and recreational activities appears to guarantee a varied experience. Yet all these variables may be held constant when participation in the wider community is compared at two different points in time. A change in the direction of less community activity, therefore, may reflect attainment of a level of adaptation similar to that of other persons in the wider community. Similarly, self-reliant behavior once manifested by retarded adults in a community facility may diminish due either to changes in residential management policy or to regression on the part of residents.

There are few case studies in which researchers have longitudinally followed mentally retarded adults relocated from state schools to community residential programs and in which changes in environment were reflected in changes in behavior.

In 1976 Birenbaum reported the results of a three-year research project in which he and Samuel Seiffer examined longitudinally what happened to a total of sixty-three men and women who left three large and isolated state schools to live at a community residence called Gatewood. Subsequent to the first report on the original cohort of sixty-three resettled persons, in April 1977 forty-two residents were still living at Gatewood. Some of those who left Gatewood were capable of more independent living, and others were incapable of community living without constant supervision. Of the twenty-one who had left, four had gone to live with their families, one moved into the community, four were participating in an apartment-living program, one was in a nursing home because of physical problems, one had voluntarily returned to a state school, nine had been returned to their state schools because of behavior unacceptable to the staff, and one had been killed by a car.

Gatewood residents were volunteers selected from three institutions serving a metropolitan area. Screening took place at the state schools, and persons who had a history of violent behavior requiring medical care beyond oral medication, and/or were regarded as incapable of either entering competitive employment, achieving sheltered-workshop status, or attending a day-center program in the community, were not considered. The people who moved to Gatewood had a mean age of 33 years. There were twice as many men as women, and many had lived in a state school for most of their lives. Their mean age at the time of admission to the state school was 15 years, 8 months (15-8), and the mean number of years in residence was 17-8. Before placement in state schools, one-half of the population had been in classes for the educable mentally retarded. All residents had been tested at state schools during the previous ten years, and their mean IQ was 50.8. All persons selected for Gatewood were able to walk, bathe, toilet, dress, and feed themselves. One-third of the population had some medical condition, and 16 percent were subject to seizures and were receiving anticonvulsant medication when transferred to the community residence. By virtue of the ethnic composition of the region at the time of admission to state schools, the predominant groups at Gatewood were Jewish (27 percent), Hispanic (26 percent), black (20 percent), and other whites (27 percent).

This study was designed to determine whether changes in self-image, interpersonal relationships, work experience, use of leisure time, personal decision-making, and social competency occurred as a result of living in a new environment. Interviews were conducted on three occasions with the 48 respondents who remained at Gatewood for at least sixteen months. The first interview took place during the week of arrival to obtain a picture of past experiences and activities at state schools; the second interview occurred seven to ten months later to determine the extent to which residents' lives had changed; the third interview was conducted after sixteen to twenty months to gain further data on their lives. Additional data were collected through 65 hours of field observation and have been presented in a discussion of the origins of Gatewood and its emergent social organization (see Birenbaum and Seiffer). A fourth interview took place with 43 respondents between forty to forty-four months after resettlement, and the results were compared with those of the third interview to determine whether any further changes had occurred in residents' reactions to community living, relations with peers and staff, and involvement in the wider community. All interviews, which were based on 52 questions, were conducted privately by a research project interviewer; each interview was taped and averaged 30 minutes in length.

Birenbaum and Seiffer reported that the people of Gatewood not only approved of their new lifestyles, but wanted to acquire even more independence. Living at Gatewood and learning to work in vocational rehabilitation programs at sheltered workshops permitted more conventional activities and greater involvement in adult activities than had been possible in their past situations. Although they become more self-reliant and developed more-personalized social relationships with their peers, they still remained dependent on the staff for many services that they probably could have learned to perform themselves. Most evident was the general lack of skills in traveling to distant locales (other than traveling to workshops), nor could they master the logistics of determining when scheduled events took place, when to leave for them, and how to get there. In this area of living, they maintained their dependence on Gatewood staff.

Did this enthusiasm for community living remain? Did the pattern of increased personalization of living that had accompanied relocation from state schools continue? Was the same degree of self-reliance maintained, increased, or decreased both where residents lived and in the wider community?

The study of community adaptation of mentally retarded adults owes much to Edgerton's pioneering work. His followup study, aptly subtitled "Years Later," indicated that stigma management was no longer a problem for most of his respondents. More important were changes in the macroenvironment, including the greater availability of public assistance for the general population during periods of economic recession. Whereas participation in work had been an indication of competence in the early 1960s, Edgerton later reported that "many of these people appear to define themselves as normal despite their lack of vocational success." Recent conceptualization in this area has obscured the fact that in some places community care has been practiced for years. In reporting on one large institution in Canada, deSilva and Fuflak wryly noted that "residents have been demitted since the facility opened in 1961 and at a progressively increasing rate." Despite the enthusiasm for the concept of normalization and the generation of manuals on how to establish and administer managed communities, adaptations by retarded adults to the community may fluctuate. It follows that the macrosocial and microsocial environments in which mentally retarded adults are placed may be subject to changes that influence behavior.

Method

The 42 residents who remained at Gatewood for almost four years were reinterviewed privately with previously asked standardized questions. All interviews in this wave were conducted by a female interviewer who was not previously known to the respondents. All interview schedules had fixed-alternative answers, since the purpose of the study was to compare the results with previous findings. All interviews were tape-recorded, and answers were checked against the interviewer's scoring to ensure accuracy. Responses were coded according to categories established for earlier interviews and discussed in detail by Birenbaum and Seiffer.

The goal of providing a longitudinal report of deinstitutionalized residents dictated the methods employed in analyzing the data. Since the major questions were whether change in behavior and attitudes continued in the resettled population, the results were compared with all responses of all residents interviewed at the three other times, rather than only the residents who remained at Gatewood for all four interviews. This comparison was made to make it more difficult to demonstrate statistically significant differences and because there was no clear direction in sample mortality. The nine returnees to state schools left Gatewood long before the third-wave interview, and the results of the comparisons with the fourth wave cannot be accounted for by their absence from the sample. On the other hand, results could be biased in the other direction, since the most able residents, and perhaps those who were most active in the community, left Gatewood to rejoin their families or participate in an apartment-living program. Comparisons of group data from the third- and fourth-wave interviews, however, demonstrated extremely strong differences in community activity, indicating that the absence of the most-independent residents could not account for these results. Moreover, the most substantial reduction was found in the category of staff-led activities.

Results

Attitudes toward community living remained favorable, but the respondents mentioned dissatisfaction more readily during the fourth interview. They were questioned on their opinions about Gatewood and scored according to whether they mentioned anything they liked or disliked. After three years at the facility, 90 percent of the respondents still mentioned favorable aspects of living at Gatewood; more than 60 percent mentioned things they did not like.

When asked how they felt about living there, positive expressions were almost identical with those expressed during third-wave interviews. A typical response was, "I like it because I have friends." There were more negative responses and fewer neutral responses during fourth-wave interviews. Most significant, no one was reluctant to complain about living conditions. Residents felt at home even when not fully satisfied with their living conditions or fellow residents: "There's nothing here but a bunch of old maids—they just fuss and pick."

Few residents contrasted their lives at Gatewood with their lives at state schools. While freedom and independence were mentioned in the second- and third-wave interviews as central features of living, activities at Gatewood and work at vocational rehabilitation settings were not mentioned when residents answered questions about what they liked. Negative comments focused around fighting, a complaint prominent in all the interviews.

Similarly, positive comments about staff members were elicited at both third- and fourth-wave interviews. Residents commented on the friendly staff, yet regarded them as being incapable of helping to reduce undesired behavior in others, a radical change in definition from mean or punitive, as they had been described when state schools were discussed during the first-wave interviews.

When they had been interviewed in 1975, residents reported desires to live on their own, and these desires had so increased that by the fourth-wave interview, 57 percent wanted to live elsewhere. While 21 percent wanted to live with their families and 10 percent wanted to be in a foster family care unit, as in the past, the leading choice (26 percent) was apartment living with roommates. Some previous residents who now lived in apartments were in regular contact with those who remained at Gatewood. One former resident returned every other Friday night to visit. One respondent said, "Everybody's moving. I don't want to stay here all my life." Returning to the family was considered a possibility, and most residents maintained family contact, with 67 percent reporting being visited at Gatewood and 50 percent reporting visits to their family's household. Family living was also reinforced by the examples of those who left to live with family. New living arrangements, therefore, remained plausible future events in the lives of the residents. Even complaints about Gatewood were based on the lack of independence, rather than on poor treatment or not getting along with fellow residents.

We had anticipated that moving from a state school to a community residence would create more opportunities to get to know fellow residents on a personal basis. The residents' social networks at the state school were compared with those at Gatewood by questions about their daily rounds of life. Residents were asked to talk about occasions or activities rather than about friends, so they would not give socially desirable answers. Only when respondents voluntarily mentioned a specific name or introduced the term "my friend" to refer to a specific individual were the answers regarded as personalized interaction. When respondents said they ate with "everybody," "anybody," or "the other residents," their answers were coded separately. Some increased personalization of activities was discerned to have taken place when the state school was compared to Gatewood concerning such matters as with whom people ate or had fun. In the fourth-wave interviews, however, about 14 percent fewer named specific people with whom they ate meals; only 19 percent named people with whom they ate. Of those who said they had fun at Gatewood, 42 percent (vs. 37 percent) mentioned specific people, either residents or staff. Neither of these changes was statistically significant.

By the time of the third-wave interview, 80 percent of the residents were attending a sheltered workshop, and two people were competitively employed. This distribution prevailed at the time of the fourth-wave interview. The workshop continued to be a source of pride and a place where an active social life was available to residents. Residents who reported having boyfriends or girlfriends often mentioned that they met them at the workshop; a slight majority, however, had found their sweethearts at Gatewood. The workshop seemed to be a more active place for sociability than in earlier interviews, with 56 percent admitting they talked while working, compared with only 40 percent two years previously. Field observations reported by Birenbaum and Seiffer indicated that the workshop experience had become a central life interest. An earlier interview with the director of a large sheltered workshop program indicated that Gatewood residents were active participants in the program's social life. This increase in conversation may have resulted from having made friends at the shop plus being able to be productive while talking. In general, respondents felt at home at their workshops: "I talk to the employees when I'm not busy. Sometimes I work and talk at the same time." While residents perceived the individual staff members of Gatewood as benign and there was little fear of punishment expressed, there was a noted shift toward greater regulation of daily living. In 1975, 60 percent of the residents had reported no negative consequences for staying up late (see Table 12.1). Now only 33 percent reported the same. Personal consequences, such as being late for work or missing breakfast, increased. Punishments from staff also increased when these two time periods are compared ($x^2 = 6.1$, 2 df, p < .03).

Respondents were also asked questions concerning who made decisions about bedtime hours and the time to get up in the morning. In 1975, respondents had reported that they were much more likely to make these decisions themselves than they had at state schools. Other similar decisions also appeared to be more in the hands of residents, such as when to get haircuts and when to take showers; however, trends toward increased responsibility and self-reliance found earlier were slightly reversed in the 1977 interviews. The residents were still more or less in charge of personal hygiene, bedtime, and waking decisions, even though failures to conform to schedules were being taken more seriously by the staff.

Because Gatewood was designed to reintegrate mentally retarded adults from state schools into the fabric of community life, it is essential to examine the extent to which residents used the community, through outings sponsored by the Gatewood staff and, even more important, through self-initiated activities. To avoid characterizing Gatewood as merely a

Table 12.1   Percentage of Residents Who Reported Consequences of Staying Up Late at Gatewood

| | Interview | |
Consequences	Third wave[a]	Fourth wave[b]
Staying up late permitted and no after-effect reported.	60	33
Staying up late permitted, but personal consequences incurred (late for work, missing breakfast)	12	23
Staying up late not permitted, and staff punish those who violate the rule.	28	44

[a] After 16 to 20 months in residence (N = 40).
[b] After 40 to 44 months in residence (N = 40).

"mini-institution," it was essential to look for evidence of the independent use of the community. During the third interview, respondents were asked whether they had engaged in any of 13 activities or gone to establishments outside Gatewood during the three previous months. A range of activities and establishments was chosen to include some that lent themselves to mass performance and others that were more conducive to individualized participation (see Table 12.2). The items were chosen to represent some of the conventional types of behavior adults in the urban environment might engage in while searching for diversions, companionship, or entertainment. If respondents reported engaging in an activity, a followup question was asked to determine whether they had attended by themselves, with another nonstaff person (most likely a peer), or with a Gatewood staff member.

In 1975 residents had reported having gone to an average of 7.4 places out of the 13 possible choices, as can be seen in Table 12.3. The most frequently mentioned were within walking distance of Gatewood—the store, the park, and the church. The residents had been encouraged to use these locations when relocated at Gatewood because of their proximity to the residence. The least frequently mentioned activities were trips to social settings where entry is somewhat restricted, such as parties, bars, and restaurants. For example, fewer than one-third of Gatewood residents reported attending parties outside the residence.

It was expected that with the passage of time greater familiarity with the wider community would occur and, therefore, residents would use it with

Table 12.2   Percentage of Gatewood Residents Attending Outside Activity and the Form of Participation

Location or activity	Interview		x^2 (1 df)
	Third wave[a]	Fourth wave[b]	
Store	94	64	10.38*
Park	83	12	45.71*
Church	75	74	2.6
Zoo	73	5	42.98*
Movies	64	36	7.47**
Parents	60	50	1.0
Restaurant	58	21	12.60*
Museum	54	12	17.71*
Friends	48	12	13.55*
Ballgame	42	5	14.58*
Community center	33	2	14.00*
Party	31	2	10.87*
Bar	23	14	.10
Other	16	1/	3.27

[a] After 16 to 20 months in residence (N = 48).
[b] After 40 to 44 months in residence (N = 42).
*p < .0001.
**p < .0004.

Table 12.3   Mean Number of Activities Undertaken by Respondents, Alone, with Others, and with Staff

Variable	Interview		t^c
	Third wave[a]	Fourth wave[b]	
Number of activities	7.4	3.14	−4.97*
Number alone	2.5	1.6	−2.86***
Number with others (fellow residents, friends relatives)	1.6	.98	−2.19**
Number with staff	3.2	.6	−5.23*

[a] After 16 to 20 months in residence (N = 48).
[b] After 40 to 44 months in residence (N = 42).
[c] Wilcoxen test for correlated data.
*p < .00001.
**p < .02.
***p < .004.

greater frequency. This expectation was not fulfilled. Gatewood residents mentioned only a mean of 3.14 activities per person (t = -4.97, p < .0001). The total volume of activities had dropped off sharply by the fourth interview. Now only visits to parents, the store, and the church remained activities in which at least half the respondents reported having taken part during the previous three months. Whereas the mean number of activities undertaken in the company of staff members was 3.2 in 1975, that average had decreased to .60 in 1977 (t = -5.23, p < .0001). As can be seen from these data, these staff-accompanied trips had not been replaced by solo ventures or journeys with peers.

In addition to the systematically elicited responses to questions concerning these activities and establishments in the wider community, respondents were asked if they ever went anywhere on their days off. Of the twenty Gatewood residents who reported excursions, twelve went by public transportation. Few residents ventured out at night; 83 percent spent their time watching television, listening to records, taking care of their rooms, or engaging in personal hygiene. One respondent commented: "I go to my niece's with my sister. There are a lot of drug addicts there. It looks like World War II hit the area. It's a disgrace."

Discussion

Revisiting Gatewood has raised many new questions about managed communities and the concept of normalization. First, it is important to note that for these mentally retarded people who had left large and isolated state schools and had lived at a community residence for almost four years, a direction of movement from dependency to greater self-reliance was not found. The period of personal exploration and the acquisition of new experiences that initially accompanied resettlement had given way to a prosaic routine of sleep, work, and at-home recreation of a passive nature; weekends were often reserved for visiting family or receiving visits. This lifestyle differs little from those who are not retarded, but are marginally employed or mostly unemployed. The discretionary income available for people on public assistance limits outings or the appropriate apparel for enjoying public places in a respectable manner.

In addition, for many city dwellers who feel vulnerable or are overly influenced by the mass media, travel at night is full of danger. Since Gatewood residents work all day on weekdays, daytime travel is largely restricted to weekends.

Second, a managed community encourages the physical separation of places of work from sleep and recreation and is still a more-conventional way of living than life in a state school or developmental center; however, privacy can limit the benefits of developing group standards of conformity and nonconformity found earlier. Furthermore, the development of informal norms could reduce the need for staff control over bedtime hours.

Third, community location and easy access to mass transportation cannot, by themselves, produce greater participation in the community beyond the world of work. One can argue that deinstitutionalized mentally retarded adults are simply becoming like everyone else and have acquired attitudes toward travel that are appropriate for a "dangerous community." Yet it was also found that residents had increased their aspirations for independent living and wished to join that community. With this in mind, it is possible that the sharp reduction of outside activity was only temporary. Moreover, there was some variability among the forms of community activity, with the sharpest reduction found among those activities led by staff members.

It is evident that if the concept of normalization is applied literally, the residents of Gatewood would earn high marks for settling into comfortable and conventional routines. As may be inferred from the interviews and from conversations with the director, Gatewood staff members stressed conformity to house rules and may have discouraged, without actually forbidding, frequent use of the wider community for entertainment and recreation. The data, however, do not explain the evident reduction of outside activity solely on the basis of a policy shift with greater restraints placed on residents by facility staff. Another explanation is that the respondents were not competent to engage in these community activities, could not continue them, and therefore regressed.

It should be cautioned that Gatewood is not a typical community residence. It is larger in size than the usual group residence. It was intended only as an early alternative to a large state school before many smaller residential settings could be developed. Therefore, data concerning Gatewood residents may not be generalizable to other community settings. Nevertheless, it would be interesting to test, by controlled longitudinal studies where social environments could be deliberately altered for mentally retarded adults randomly assigned to several types of community-based programs, the alternative hypothesis that the various inadequacies of the residents themselves cause the changes in behavior over time.

13

Mutual Aid Support Among Mentally Retarded Adults Living in Apartments

Introduction

This chapter describes the informal mutual aid for and counseling among twenty-seven male and six female mentally retarded adults living in widely dispersed apartments, more than half of whom relocated from state schools. Living alone (22 percent) or with roommates (78 percent) in apartments and without direct supervision was a new experience for the residents, who had an average IQ of 62.4 and averaged 33.4 years of age. Ethnically, the study group was 72 percent white, 19 percent Hispanic and 9 percent black. These persons were monitored by the community care staff of Bronx Developmental Services, a community-based service agency.

At the time of this study, residents had lived in their apartments for an average of 18 months. Supplemental Security Income (81 percent) and public assistance (19 percent) provided financial support for the residents. Homemaker services were available. The residents spent the majority of their days participating in sheltered workshops to earn pocket money (51 percent), engaged in competitive employment at close to minimum wages (24 percent), participating in the New York City Board of Education's Occupational Training Center programs (7 percent), or neither working nor in any day programs (18 percent).

The concept of the need for psychosocial support is not new to the field of mental retardation. The role of the "benefactor" has been identified as supportive of newly deinstitutionalized mentally retarded adults. Often the person who plays the role of the "benefactor" is a neighbor or employer, indicating some concern on the part of the mentally retarded to avoid stigmatizing agency contacts. Support can be provided by a psychosocial network of neighbors and friends. How do these informal networks develop, especially when counseling and supervision are also supplied by a developmental center's community services staff?

Data Collection Techniques

Other research investigations have found that mentally retarded adults regarded researchers as part of the staff available to solve their problems, especially when no agency staff members were on hand. Therefore, home visitation by researchers may have discouraged independent problem solving, and there was no observation of daily living in the home.

Since data on mutual aid in our study of apartment living arrangements could not always be learned from the behavior and statements of participants at scheduled group meetings, research had to include more than observation of programmed activities. Furthermore, some self-sufficient members of the program rarely attended the instructional group sessions. Staff reported that members who did not attend group meetings (more than half the residents) fell into two categories: isolates with few informal social relationships who depended strictly on staff for the solution of major problems (e.g., regaining lost SSI benefits), and those clients depending almost exclusively on informal social support.

To learn how the program members managed those problems that were not recounted, each was given a ten-question open-ended interview. They were asked to tell how they would solve recurrent daily problems so other people could benefit from their experience. Problems were based mainly on situations requiring either the help of another person or an extension of help on the respondent's part to someone else, and the responses were considered to be indirect indicators of the adaptive behavior of mentally retarded adults living in apartments. Answers were also used as a basis for determining whether social networks could be identified.

Interview responses were scored according to the persons from whom clients sought help in their attempt to solve the hypothetical problems; other members of the program—friends, roommates, or neighbors—earned a score of two points; relatives or family earned a score of one point; and no points were gained when staff members were indicated. All other answers also received a score of zero. When respondents named a prospective helper or companion, they were always asked to identify the person according to the categories listed above. The rationale for the scoring followed the findings in the literature on the correlation between community adaptation and social support. Answers about potential helpers were scored more highly than the second group because these social relationships were self-initiated, rather than based on family ties. Reliance on staff for the solution of minor problems was considered unnecessary and consequently was scored lower. All the situations presented to respondents were designed to determine strategies employed in apartment living and were hypothetical. Some respondents even volunteered that similar situations had, in fact, arisen recently.

Observation of the interactions between clients and staff was another method used to collect data. It was anticipated that many of the difficulties encountered and the strategies employed to cope by the mentally retarded adults would be expressed in the regularly scheduled group meetings with staff and the other residents. Over a period of six months, thirty hours of undisguised observation took place at the main offices of the apartment living program. During these occasions, staff instructed members about many of the activities of daily living such as cleaning, measuring units used in cooking, and marketing. In addition, clients discussed the following concerns about the apartment living experiences with peers and staff: how to fix up and maintain an apartment, how to deal with landlords and superintendents, and how to manage relationships with staff homemakers and roommates. At these meetings, clients identified instances of informal mutual aid when recounting how they solved day-to-day problems without staff intervention.

Findings

For these mentally retarded adults, community life involved many new experiences and problems. A generic difficulty focused on the question of how to get along with roommates. Staff counseling efforts reduced conflict between roommates, but when roommates were assigned it always involved staff intervention, not merely approval. In general, clients were reluctant to call upon fellow program members for help with major problems.

With or without the assistance of roommates, moving into his own apartment was an unprecedented experience in the life of each mentally retarded adult. Along with cleaning and fixing up an apartment, the transportation of furniture and clothing was a considerable task. Initially, members of the program were reluctant to call upon each other for help; staff needed to ask for help for them. Prior living experiences in state schools had provided no counterpart, since most major tasks there had been initiated and completed under direct staff supervision. Similarly, living with kin apparently provided little opportunity or need to help or be helped by friends or neighbors.

Client-staff relations were a source of pride at the apartment living program. Staff members acknowledged the strength of these ties as a way of keeping a kindly watch over clients in the community. In turn, clients used these ties to get things done, as when staff often assisted clients to arrange for help from fellow clients in moving. However, staff did not use these same strong ties to teach social skills to prevent future interventions. Major problems of community living, such as moving, occur more than once in a lifetime; and asking for help is a learned skill that can be used often in the course of a lifetime of any individual.

Living in the community for most clients involved contact with the staff at evening programs. Clients who attended these programs were also observed interacting cooperatively with each other at the offices of the apartment living program. Nevertheless, client behavior was more socially appropriate in the company of staff than in the company of fellow clients. Perhaps it was status enhancing for clients to spend time talking to staff (or be seen doing so); in any case, clients preferred to be with staff rather than their peers. In contrast to Edgerton's population, program members who appeared for evening activities were not stigmatized by agency contact.

On a groupwide basis, other problems of daily living were less easy to identify. Securing employment most often required staff intervention, although some members did query other residents about openings where they worked. Members of the program also shared emotional support as well as information. One of the most socially skilled members of the program actively encouraged other men to meet and enjoy the company of women at a dance scheduled by the agency. Finally, a few friendships were noted to exist beyond staff-assigned roommates.

From these data three questions emerged that are related to social networks and how they are used:

1. Do members of the program claim to rely on staff or others to solve day-to-day problems that require thoughtful planning to achieve goals?
2. When program members do rely on people other than staff to solve serious problems, are those helping individuals people who live close by or far away?
3. Are specific subgroups identified in the pattern of aid between clients and others? Do reciprocal choices exist as to whom one goes for help?

Answers to these questions will provide some basis for determining both the importance of informal social support in the lives of the respondents and patterns of utilization.

All the clients were presented with hypothetical dilemmas, scored as noted earlier. Total dependence on staff led to a minimum score of zero, while total dependence on other program members, friends, and neighbors resulted in a maximum score of twenty. Dependence on staff for help was relatively infrequent. Of the total of 330 answers from all respondents, staff were relied on for help in only 10 percent of the cases. As can be seen in Table 13.1, staff were most heavily requested for help to solve four problems: moving furniture, party arrangements, first aid, and lost keys. Even in those four categories, those who would call upon staff for help constituted no more than one-third of the clients.

These data were correlated with the IQ score of the respondent, the number of months he had lived in an apartment, and his age. Little variance could be accounted for by these independent variables. Sociometric techniques disclosed seven distinct groups of three or more people not linked to each other. Indicators for groups were based on the naming, as prospective helpers or companions, of neighbors who were not members of the program, or members naming each other. This method of establishing the existence of groups is based on patterns of interaction assumed to exist beyond the solution of hypothetical problems. All persons named always lived within three or four city blocks of the respondent.

Table 13.1   Hypothetical Questions Asked of 33 Mentally Retarded Adults Living in Apartments, and Their Responses

Where problem has serious consequences for respondent	Choice of Answer				Total score
	Staff	Family	Other	No answer	
*1. If you needed something from the supermarket,but you couldn't go out, is there anyone who could bring something back for you? If yes, who?	2	3	23	5	49
*2. If you were going away but you were expecting a delivery, are there any people who could take in the package while you were away? If yes, who?	2	3	22	6	47
3. If you lost your keys to your apartment on a weekend, where would you stay?	7	6	16	4	38
4. Someone is willing to give you a couch for your apartment. It is in the building where you live but you need help to move it. Is there anyone you could ask to help you move it into your apart-ment? If yes. who?	10	2	18	3	38
5. You cut your hand and need someone to help you with the bandage. Who would you ask?	8	0	17	8	34
6. Lots of people lend things to other people. And lots of people don't. Have you ever lent some-thing to anyone since you started living on your own? If yes, who?	1	0	17	15	34
*7. Your TV is broken and you want to watch your favorite program. Is there anyone you could talk to about getting a chance to watch at	1	2	23	7	48

Table 13.1 cont.

Where problem has serious consequences for respondent	Choice of Answer				Total score
	Staff	Family	Other	No answer	
their house? If yes, who?					
8. If someone gave you two free tickets for a show, what would you do with the extra ticket?	1	2	23	8	48
9. If you wanted to go to the movies on a Satur-day, would you go alone or call someone? If you call someone, who would it be?	2	2	18	11	38
10. You want to have a party but you don't know how many people to invite. Is there anyone who could help you figure this out? If yes, who?	8	0	17	8	34

* Where assistance from people living nearby is most appropriate to solve the problem.

Conclusions

Informal local groups emerged that were formed not only of some members of the apartment living program per se, but also of some program members, neighbors, and friends. In addition, hypothetical dilemmas requiring help from others were solved without naming staff members in 84 percent of the appropriate answers. How much of this outcome can be explained by the efforts of staff? Some of the members of the program attended classes and workshops designed to improve their adaptive skills, yet some of the most independent and interdependent members of the groups were rarely seen at the office.

Logically, people with limited financial resources and time should develop local contacts for acquiring social support. Following that assumption, mentally retarded adults who are part of an apartment living program might also use nearby human resources to compensate for their lack of material resources. People who live nearby may be used as personal benefactors, a role played by neighbors and employers in the lives of the mentally retarded adults studied by Edgerton.

In a community that lacks material resources, the mentally retarded adult may be seen by neighbors as a source of help. If his apartment has a complete set of cleaning implements and kitchenware, he may be called upon to share the scarce resources. This enables the mentally retarded adult to trade favors. A similar pattern is identified among elderly people in poor neighborhoods. Elderly who receive social security checks may be viewed as good people to know by those without steady incomes, and with whom sharing a household makes good sense. Similarly, mentally retarded adults may be accorded prestige for what they own and can trade; therefore, they may be less subject to social derogation for being incompetent.

Staff deliberately located the younger and more capable clients a greater distance from the main office than those who needed more supervision and an easier commute. Being some distance from the main office of an apartment living program appears to encourage mutual aid, rather than dependence on staff, for assistance in the problems of daily living. Since money is scarce, a client's travel to see his counselor may be curtailed and he may learn to solve problems without official involvement. Nonetheless, staff finds too much independence a matter of concern because it makes it difficult for them to assess how clients are managing.

Informal social support groups can be purposely shaped through a combination of a scarcity of resources and the physical distance from the office. Staff can selectively utilize apartments that are neither clustered around a centralized office nor convenient to public transportation to foster mutual aid. Therefore, community placement and deinstitutionalization for mentally retarded adults can be manipulated for the benefit of all concerned. A variety of social relationships can be engendered similar to those existing among ordinary people in the community. Apartment living can be another step in returning mentally retarded adults into the mainstream of the neighborhood.

14

Family Care Providers: Sources of Role Strain and its Management

Foster care in volunteer families has become a routine way of providing community care for mentally retarded persons. The success of such programs depends, in the final analysis, upon the quality of care provided by the family. Their performance, in turn, reflects a number of factors, such as material resources provided by the supervisory agency. Less visible but important factors affecting performance are relations with the agency personnel, the nature of foster parents' interaction with the client placements and their natural parents, and contacts within the family of the provider of care.

Maintaining placements in foster care homes depends on successful management or resolution of three ongoing sources of stress faced by foster family caretakers for mentally retarded children and, to a lesser extent, adults. Stress emerges from (a) derogation by members of the community for the person who voluntarily assumes the care of stigmatized persons, (b) the difficulty in measuring "sufficiency" when caring for a handicapped person with limited ability, and (c) the incongruence found in submitting parental discretion to agency supervision. This chapter focuses on the caretaker role and its stresses and identifies techniques of coping by its performers.

Most of the focus in the literature on foster or family care is on the potentially traumatic situations forced upon the foster child; few articles deal with the dilemmas faced by the foster parents. Some reports have covered the ambiguous role and self-definitions given to or derived by foster care parents themselves; some investigators have considered how social workers negotiate the difficult relationships among natural parents, foster parents, and foster children; and, quite appropriately, a large body of literature has emerged on how to select foster parents. While impressionistic evidence suggests that there are problematic features inherent in the family care provider role, few empirically based analyses have been attempted. More important, the study of the way family care is provided for mentally retarded children and adults has been largely ignored. What follows is an examinination of how uncertainties and ambiguities built into the role of family care provider produce stresses and strains for the performer.

Why should the expectations associated with a role be a source of strain? Tension is created in reference to any role in that its performance reflects on the performer. This predicament is not merely a question of good or bad performance; the very fulfillment of role obligations involves relations with others (preceding and simultaneous with incumbency), activities that produce discrepancies between what is and what ought to be, between past and present, and between idealized standards and real behavior. Performing a role implies evaluation by others, often referred to by sociologists as social status. If status is something conferred by others, and each role performed is evaluated by others, then personal relationships and bonds between people are sources of role strain. In fact, sometimes the more skillfully one performs, particularly socially derogated roles, the worse personal relations become with others. Alternatively, persons accorded high status may give up roles that detract from their image.

Interviews with twenty caretakers associated with Bronx Developmental Services (BDS) provide evidence about the common role problems and their solutions that affect foster parents for the developmentally disabled. A random sample of nineteen females and one male was administered an extensive schedule of 51 open-ended questions in privately conducted taped interviews of approximately 35 minutes. Since our concern was with techniques developed by performers of the family care role to deal with ongoing dilemmas, it was appropriate to derive findings from self-reports on their achievements, rather than to use objective measures of performance. Successful role performance is related to developing cognitive mechanisms for the manipulation or redefinition of stressful situations. Findings are presented according to the three ongoing problems faced in providing family care to the developmentally disabled.

Voluntarily Caring for a Stigmatized Individual

Foster care candidates, like all persons voluntarily applying to fill roles, can be understood in terms of the widely recognized behavioral pattern of seeking the most esteemed or high-status roles available. The family care provider role is clearly among the most attractive available to the population from which most BDS applicants come, that is, one characterized by lower education and income levels and minority status. For such individuals the selection and certification for this role by a largely middle-class bureaucracy is in itself a status-enhancing experience, and the compensation for their services is an important incentive. In addition, certain segments of the community at large, such as church and civic groups, view the performance of the foster care role favorably, which contributes to increased self-esteem and prestige.

The assumption of the family care provider role is not viewed in a positive light by everyone, however. As McCoy (1962a) notes, while some segments of the community define foster parents as "virtuous," others look on these role performers with "suspicion." Compounding one's relations with the larger community is the fact that developmentally disabled clients are themselves looked upon with "suspicion."

Various terms have been used by social scientists to describe the attribution of less-than-human or non-normal characteristics to the population served by our respondents. While society's detrimental view of their clients might, at face value, not appear to be a problem for caretakers themselves, this is not the case. As persons "related through the structure to the stigmatized individual," Goffman (1963) reminds us, they are "obliged to share some of the discredit," since stigma tends to "spread out in waves." In other words, to use Goffman's term, family care providers, because of their being "afforded courtesy membership in the clan," have to contend with "courtesy stigma," a labeling by society leading both the stigmatized and those associated with them to be "treated...as one." Furthermore, Goffman suggests that relations between the nonstigmatized and the courtesy stigmatized "tend either to be avoided or to be terminated." It is conceivable, moreover, that these foster parents are doubly stigmatized— first, because of their intimate association with stigmatized persons and, second, because of the voluntary nature of their association.

Given, therefore, that relations with stigmatized persons are generally avoided, how do we account for foster parents who voluntarily choose to associate with persons who will inevitably be responsible for their being negatively affected by "courtesy stigma"?

Social derogation can be managed through association with respectable people. The increased status and prestige forthcoming from the agency and segments of the community do alleviate or counteract some of the negative effects of courtesy stigma. In addition, the caretakers' definition of their role as designed to serve a worthy social purpose, as clearly indicated in professed motivations and satisfactions (whether a religious or social conscience orientation), helps to cast what to some may be a "disvalued" or "disrespectable" position in a positive light. Increased senses of self-esteem and religious motivations, however, are of themselves inadequate to resolve this source of role strain. Additional techniques must be developed by caretakers if they are to feel comfortable in a clearly problematic situation. Family care providers revealed three basic techniques they employed to deal with this potential loss of respectability.

First, since roles imply relationships and are therefore reciprocal, how caretakers define their clients is of great importance for their personal role definitions. Therefore, it is not surprising that the basic coping mechanism identified involves foster parents' attempts to convince themselves that the differences between their clients and normal children are minimal, hence eliminating the primary cause of their having been labeled other than "respectable."

> Normal or retarded—they *all* have the *same problems*. The *only* difference is
> they can't *grasp* things so readily. Only after I went to *class* I knew that two kids
> I had care for [in a day care program] were retarded. [Emphasis in original.]

Of course, this suspension of belief in and of itself is obviously inadequate to counteract their clients', and subsequently their own, culturally imposed deviant status. Foster care parents are all too aware of the differences between their placements and "fully human" (to use Goffman's phrase) children, as now noted, "To *me* they're *not* retarded. . . . I know *inside* they're retarded though."

Second, family care providers try to avoid relationships, situations, or encounters that highlight or reinforce their "differentness." In their quest for a "normal-appearing round of life," respondents strictly limit their association with other family care providers and tend to avoid participation in purposive foster parents groups, a pattern similarly characterizing natural mothers of retarded children.

Finally, some family care providers adopt a professional, active approach to dealing with the stigmatizing condition. Caretakers tend to engage in some form of a consciousness-raising campaign, directly attacking society's imposition of the deviant label on their foster children. What this educational aspect of the role actually entailed varied among our respondents, whose remarks ran the gamut from those of the dispassionate teacher to the ideological crusader. A small number of respondents did interpret the role as having as its goal the preparation of clients for independent living (or at least greatly increased participation) within the community context. As two respondents commented: "I teaches them to be independent, travel, shop and do for their own." And "*They* should belong in society *too*...why *not*?" To others, however, the "community" consisted solely of a protective family unit, where "one of the family" was defined as the only community role the child could be expected to, or was permitted to, play. Because they view their role as including the shielding of the client from hostile outsiders, some parents unfortunately prevented clients' development of relationships with supportive others.

The Notion of "Sufficient Effort" in a Parenting Role

The second source of role strain we will discuss is the uncertainty faced by foster parents in determining what constitutes adequate role performance. What levels of effort, commitment, and investment are required to successfully fulfill their duties and responsibilities toward their client, and at least as important, what do caretakers perceive as the *agency's* definition of "sufficiency"?

The resolution of this uncertainty requires that family care providers develop a personal notion of role-appropriate attitudes and behavior, that is, a role definition or conception. A lack of role clarity will, it is assumed, become a source of impaired functioning for the role incumbent. Yet the development of a family caretaker role conception is problematic. Indeed, Ambinder and his colleagues found that nearly half their sample were unable to provide a working definition of their role. This difficulty arises for several reasons. First, unlike most role incumbents, family care providers do not have much chance to learn about and practice their roles (even by exposure to media and educational experiences of relevance) before they assume the position themselves. Nor do they have much opportunity to interact with other similarly positioned individuals prior to their certification. Second, because of the preference of our respondents not to associate with other caretakers after entry into the position, a functioning network that might provide feedback, social support, and normative instruction has been unable to develop. Third, foster parents receive only limited formal training in preparation for their assumption of this new position. What they do receive more closely resembles an orientation. Fourth, the agency has not established formal requirements for performance of caretaking duties other than those related to minimal health and safety standards; rather, only general guidelines exist.

The last two reasons are not the result of a shortcoming on the part of the agency: they reflect the undeniable difficulty of defining the family care provider role. Davids has observed that "foster care parenting is not a stable, regular work situation...[T]he requirements of the role change with the child's needs." Simply, the foster parent role requires flexibility for successful performance, and this flexibility gives rise to ambiguous responses to the family care provider, which can be the source of considerable personal tension and strain, in addition to impaired role performances.

Despite these difficulties, some conception of a role's required duties and attitudes must precede its assumption. Family care providers, for the most part, conceptualize their role as analogous to that of a natural parent. Indeed, without a parental orientation these providers would not be selected by the agency. Remarks such as the following identify the "mothering" role orientation and suggest its importance in the role definition process:

He [the client] really *needs* me. He's my baby even though he's 12 years old.

My kids [the clients know that] underneath the Christmas tree there's a present *whatever* the group gives them or not. I give them T.L.C. I treat them *better* than their own parents.

I feel *lost* if I don't have children around. It was a *must* for me to have a child.

When asked what they, as individuals, had to offer the clients, four specifically mentioned "being a mother to them." "Giving love" was cited by an additional six. Three foster mothers believed that their foster children would never be reunited with their natural parents for the simple reason that the clients preferred to remain with them, whom they considered their "real mothers." Clearly, then, the "mothering" parallel figures prominently in family care providers' definitions of their roles as the primary model for performance.

It is altogether reasonable that foster parents have chosen to rely upon a parenting model of behavior. One rationale for this perspective, sometimes stated explicitly and sometimes implicitly by our respondents, is that the most critical factor responsible for their selection and certification was their success in raising their own natural families. In fact, family care providers repeatedly justified their initial and continued performance of the role on the ground that their perception of the role's primary responsibiity, "being a parent" to the client, meshed precisely with what they viewed as their natural talents, inclinations, and experience. They clearly defined the role requirements of their natural and foster parenting roles as similar. As two noted, "Without patience, love and time, you wouldn't make very good parents anyway," and "If they're *any* kind of parent, they'll find these things—love and time—are necessary."

Even though family care providers tend to define their roles as analogous to those of natural parents, this does not completely resolve the problem of role ambiguity. Choosing this orientation raises the very real question of the extent to which the analogy is appropriate. When this model is considered more than a heuristic device to facilitate the day-to-day negotiation of the role, role strain and conflict situations inevitably multiply. Fanshel and Shinn noted that the responsiblities of foster and natural parents are indeed equivalent. We would be mistaken, however, if we, assume an equivalence between *tasks* (aspects of the division of labor) normally performed in conjunction with a role and the *role* itself, which implies reciprocal *relationships* rather than characteristic elements of role behavior. At this point, therefore, the natural parenting analogy breaks down, for although the tasks associated with the two roles have much in common, the relationships they imply do not.

Casting oneself in the role of a parent implies that one construes of the client placement as one's child—a role the placement, the agency, or the natural parent may be unwilling for the child to play. If this important structural distinction between foster and natural parent roles is not observed or, in other words, if the natural parenting analogy is embraced too fully, various types of role strain will confront the family care provider.

Five potential sources of role strain involving the foster parent/foster child relationship may result from overreliance on the natural parenting model. These are (a) conflicts between the family care provider role and incumbents' simultaneous roles of natural parent and spouse; (b) stresses caused by the possible loss of the foster child; (c) difficulties in relying on foster children for the provision of "rewards" and satisfaction; (d) conflicts with the foster child's natural parents; and (e) problems from receiving payment for being a foster parent, i.e., for providing what in foster parents' own conception is the greatest contribution they have to offer—love. (A sixth potential source of role strain, the subjection of parental discretion to agency supervision. will be discussed later.)

CONFLICTS WITH NATURAL FAMILIES OF
FAMILY CARE PROVIDERS

Since the introduction of another person into the family system invariably
gives rise to some degree of stress, the cooperation of all family members
and their reinforcement of the natural parenting role conception are
required if the foster child is to be integrated into the family context. The
allocation of a foster parent's limited resources is at the heart of the matter.
An equitable distribution of time between natural and foster children is
essential but, as Davids indicated, it is almost impossible to achieve a
distribution acceptable to all parties. Similarly, husbands may resent their
wives devoting time to the foster child and their mothering of children not
"fathered" by themselves. In addition, husbands may consider their status
has declined in comparison to their wives' increased status resulting from
their relationships with the agency. Further, wives' successfully obtaining
this form of "employment" may further their independence of their spouses.

One technique to avoid such conflicts involves individuals organizing their
roles by priority in hierarchies, favoring the roles that provide greater
satisfaction or are subject to severe negative sanctions if neglected. There is,
of course, strong cultural pressure to favor one's roles as spouse and natural
parent, and adherence to this hierarchical arrangement lessens the frequency and severity of choices among competing obligations. This does not
imply, however, that adherence to this hierarchical arrangement of
responsibilities will completely free foster parents from stressful situations.
For example, one family care provider who wished to receive an additional
placement abandoned the idea because her natural son objected to her
intention. While she put her natural parent role first, she did not attempt to
disguise her displeasure in having to do so. In general, however, our
respondents seem to be getting the cooperation they require, if they are to
truly make the foster child feel as if he or she "belongs."

THE LOSS OF A FOSTER CHILD

The ever-present prospect that the foster child may be removed by the
natural parents or the agency is a strong deterrent to complete adoption of
the natural parent analogy. Conversely, if this analogy *is* strictly adopted, a
significant amount of role strain will be generated. Swindall observed that
the role of family care provider has an undefined time span, i.e., the foster
parent is necessarily "suspended" in the child's life. This feature has been
discussed repeatedly in light of the possible detrimental effects of turnover
in homes on the child. The other side of the coin—the stressful nature of the
experience for the foster parents—also deserves recognition.

Despite this potential difficulty, only three of our respondents had as their
goal the care and training of the child in anticipation of his or her return to
the natural family, and sixteen of the twenty could not envision a time when
their placements would ever leave their homes. Since they viewed their

foster children as almost-permanent family members, it is not surprising that the prospect of losing them was quite painful for most family care providers in our sample.

I don't even think about them going back.

I *would* [take another placement], but it *wouldn't* be the same.

I wish they [her foster children] would *always* stay with me.

I shouldn't say this. I'm a mother and would *hate* them to rip away *my* kids.

The strength and predominance of the natural parent analogy as a model for the family care provider/client relationship is perhaps more appropriate for our sample of foster parents than for caretakers of a more normal population. As Jacobs cautions, return to the natural home and adoption, the primary goals for normal children temporarily in foster care, are rarely viable alternatives for mentally retarded clients who are frequently older or whose parents are unwilling or unable to care for them. Consequently, the long-term nature of many of these placements facilitates the development of expressive and intimate relationships between foster parents and clients.

Avoidance of the development of intimate relationships with foster children is clearly not the answer to this problem, and would be dysfunctional for both client and foster parent. One remedy entails the acceptance of additional placements, which virtually every respondent in our sample was prepared to do. By shifting emphasis from the child to the agency, foster parents are able to develop, to some extent, conceptualizations of themselves not as caretaker for individual children, but rather as agents of an organization caring for needy children in general.

THE EXPECTATION OF REWARDS
FROM FOSTER CARE PLACEMENTS

The third potentially problematic situation involves role strain resulting from foster parents' expecting rewards or positive feedback from the clients served who may be unable to respond, due to their disabilities, previous difficulties with their natural parents, or as an effect of experience in an institutional setting. While the normal parent-child relationship involves the parents giving love and receiving a measure of love and respect in return, McCoy notes "only limited reciprocity" can, in all fairness, be expected from a foster child. Wilkes attributes family care providers' unrealistic expectations to their ambiguous role definitions, which makes the satisfactions that can reasonably be demanded also ephemeral. Williston suggests that to shield themselves from disappointment, foster parents should adopt a new set of expectations concerning role-related rewards—specifically, that satisfactions and positive feedback provided by the agency and the community at large should supplement, if not largely supplant, rewards expected from the client. Such a strategy has been adopted to a limited degree by our sample of family caretakers, in that they identified recognition of improvement in the child's functioning as their principal source of role satisfaction, while the development of satisfactory expressive relationships with the clients, i.e., "receiving love," was relegated to second position.

CONFLICTS IN THE NATURAL PARENT/FOSTER PARENT RELATIONSHIP

A fourth potential source of role strain associated with the adherence to a natural parenting role conceptualization results from actual or anticipated interaction with the natural parents of the foster children. Clearly, such interaction jeopardizes the foster parents' primary role conception as natural parent surrogates, and focuses attention on the ambiguous boundaries and unspecified duties appropriate to these competing role partners. One of the most potentially troublesome aspects of managing the foster parent role—the extent to which this relationship is in fact stressful—depends on the amount of interaction with the parents, how much the natural parents accept what the foster parent can do for the client, and how attached the foster parent has become to the child. Garrett suggests that "the implication of failure in the [natural] parental role" can strain foster/natural parent relations from the outset, in that confrontation with persons selected to perform a role, which another has been forced to relinquish through "failure," can sabotage the most well intentioned efforts to develop or promote a "positive" relationship.

Very little interaction—or interference—between foster and natural parents was found in our sample. Thus, role definition performance is eased, since the noninterference of natural parents accounts for one less source of role expectations and, therefore, fewer possible sources of incompatible demands that are largely responsible for the existence of role strains, conflicts, and sociologically ambivalent situations. It is clear, however, that those who do interact with their clients' natural parents encounter somewhat stressful relationships.

> One mother comes to my house to play with *my* grandson and doesn't pay attention to her *own* son. It brought tears to my eyes. He [the foster child] threw his arms around her. *Why* doesn't she love him?

Family care providers in our sample tended to mitigate this source of role strain by emphasizing the therapeutic function they performed, distinguishing themselves from natural parents without having to weigh the relative amounts of "love" given by parents and themselves to the child. Again, caretakers' emphasis on the therapeutic, professional aspects of their role, rather than the nurturing features, is a move away from the problematic natural parenting role conception and a step in the direction of the development of a distinct foster parent job description.

RECEIVING PAYMENT FOR PARENTING

The emphasis on therapeutic functions and developmental objectives is also used by family care providers to deal with the fifth source of role strain resulting from the adoption of the parenting analogy, namely, being paid for parenting. The role of the natural parent is predicated upon giving love freely and for free to one's children; however, when foster parents attempt to adopt a parenting role, they must deal with the fact that they receive monthly compensation for the love they give the child.

To resolve this incompatibility of role aspects, family caretakers focus upon their skills, certification, and training, all aspects of an occupational or professional role definition, which serve to legitimate their being compensated for their services. It is important to note however, that undertaking the family care provider role solely "for the money" met with universal condemnation from our sample. Respondents were in agreement that foster caretaking was no "ordinary job," but rather more akin to a "calling." One's "worthiness" had to be proved before he or she was selected for the position; as one respondent stated, "*Some* people don't *deserve* to have anybody!" In sum, a very high degree of commitment and personal involvement was perceived to be a necessary element of adequate role performance. Clearly, therefore, monetary reward alone could not serve as a primary inducement for the assumption of the role.

Given the similarity in foster parent/natural parent role tasks, and the importance of foster parents' previous experience as natural parents for their selection and certification, it is not surprising that family caretakers adopt a natural parent analogy as the basis for role definition. Adopting the natural parent model, however, creates new strains. While this model does provide guidance for role incumbents, it simultaneously creates several sources of role strain, all of which call attention to the fact that the natural parenting analogy is applicable only in terms of role-related tasks, not implied role relationships.

In seeking to resolve conflicts that arise in this connection, family care providers redefine their role in ways that differentiate it from that of the natural parent. To deal with the possible removal of the child and insufficient rewards received from clients, caretakers move away from the definition of the client as primary role partner and substitute the agency as the most salient reciprocal role partner. A new ideology emerges through efforts to resolve the incompatibility of being paid for parenting and the inevitable conflicts with the client's natural parents, one in which family care providers tend to emphasize their professional or therapeutic functions apart from or in addition to their duties as surrogate parents.

This is not to suggest that the natural parent role analogy has been abandoned by family care providers. To the contrary, the parenting model is clearly their primary guideline for performance. Yet its apparent inadequacies and attendant role strains lead family care providers to modify their role conceptions to accommodate those aspects of the role—particularly the foster parent-client relationships—that are incompatible with the natural parent analogy.

The Subjection of Parental Discretion
to Agency Supervision

Foster parents, in their adoption of the "natural parenting" role conception, subject themselves to an additional role strain: the subordination of a parent's primary authority over child-rearing decisions to the inspection, review, and evaluation of an overseeing agency. The agency is primarily responsible for all major decisions in the foster parenting situation. Accountability to persons other than one's immediate family clearly jeopardizes a natural-parenting role definition, which, in turn, produces stress for those operating on the basis of that model. One caretaker, dismayed at being thwarted in her attempt to exercise parental discretionary authority, a duty and right she considered to be appropriate to her definition of the role, gave vent to her frustration: "I can't feel like a real mother cause I have to call her—the case manager, call the *teacher*. . . . I feel like nothing!"

One could reasonably ask whether natural parents are, in fact, immune from outside inspection. Pressures as to when to have a child, with whom, and under what circumstances are important, although often subtle, standard considerations in social life. In additional, parents ordinarily strive to be awarded the community's label of "good, responsible parent" as an accolade with widespread ramifications for the assumption of adequate performance in other apparently unrelated roles, such as employee, political candidate, and the like. As much as natural parents admittedly do not perform their roles oblivious to outside pressures, the pressures impinging on the foster parent are clearly of a different, more controlling order. The screening of applicants to determine their suitability and, if they are certified, the subsequent continual monitoring of activities within the family setting have no parallel in the natural parent role.

The data reveal that respondents cope with the fact of agency supervision in much the same way as they deal with a role strain discussed previously (i.e., receiving financial rewards for providing "love"): they define their role as entailing more than solely nurturing aspects. Insofar as it is possible to partially conceptualize the family caretaker position as an occupation, the respondents' legitimate supervision and evaluation (like payment) are standard features of any job.

Defining their roles as incorporating "professional" features not only protects family care providers from what could be construed as a trespassing of parental rights, but it also results in their increased self-esteem because of their demonstrated expertise in child-rearing, the professional criteria on the basis of which they were certified, and their formal and on-the-job training. Their ability to be proud of their training and their having "passed" a parenting test eliminates not only role strain resulting from the ambiguity of the boundaries between natural and foster parenting, but also alleviates the role dilemma inherent in outside monitoring of what is, in general, a private affair.

It should be noted that while training experiences enable family care providers to deal with these two role strain situations, it is clear that in the eyes of family care providers training alone cannot produce a good foster parent. On the contrary, respondents primarily emphasize their natural, intrinsic capacities and talents for fostering. This sentiment was frequently expressed; for example, "Caring for kids—it must come natural!" Natural ability also meant that respondents were expert and had a monopoly on the required skill. So, while the nineteen caretakers who had been trained by Bronx Developmental Services conceded the experience had been at least moderately stimulating and useful, only five deemed it sufficient. Eleven who conceded it was a "good start" took pride in recounting instances in which they had supplemented that training with their own resourcefulness and parental skills. Foster parents' conception of their role requirements, entailing not only the professional training requisites, which legitimated their being evaluated, but also unteachable personal skills, serves two purposes: protecting role incumbents from formalized evaluations based exclusively on universalistic criteria, and enhancing their self-esteem in terms of their "specialness."

The development of a role definition that stresses the critical importance of natural talent for adequate role performance cannot completely shield foster parents from unpleasant features of agency evaluation. In dealing with this potentially stressful situation, one which could result in their loss of a valued role, caretakers attempt to transform the nature of the relationship with the agency from a possibly intimidating to a nonthreatening one. Since their involvement with their case managers constitutes, for all intents and purposes, their relationship with the agency, it is not surprising that family care providers attempt to convert their social workers to friends or confidantes. By befriending their case managers and establishing particularistic relationships with them, caretakers downplay the asymmetrical nature of the interaction between themselves and the superordinate, evaluating agency. Once such a personal bond is cemented and one's competence and commitment (the behavioral and attitudinal components of the role) are demonstrated, the ongoing process of evaluation that could otherwise be intrusive and intimidating is for the most part completed, barring any radical change in caretaking functioning, household composition, or client needs. The development of a particularistic relationship with case managers also serves the important purpose of furnishing family care providers with a functional reference group, a source of feedback and social support that is lacking because of their isolation from other foster care providers.

The appropriation of a case manager as confidante or colleague presupposes some degree of the case manager's cooperation. It appears that case managers do indeed encourage this familiar, rather than formal, relationship, because playing the role of friend makes their own duties more manageable, by freeing them from having to penetrate a screen of distrust in their attempts to serve both clients and foster parents.

Given the importance of the case manager's approval to caretakers' continuance as agents for BDS, great care is taken, by means of what are termed "impression management" techniques in Goffman's dramaturgical approach to social interaction, to aid evaluators in the formation of an opinion of caretakers' performance consonant with the impression parents hope to convey. It is essential that caretakers establish not only the observable tasks associated with the role are performed (role conte but that they are undertaken and accomplished with the proper motivati and commitment (role style).

The caretakers use a number of techniques to this end: the assumption of a sincerely intense attitude, using a highly interested and animated tone of voice while conversing with agency personnel, and the casual but deliberate presentation of "hard evidence" of exemplary role performance, such as displaying photographs of broadly smiling clients on vacation. Data collected from BDS evaluators themselves revealed the importance of an applicant's "apparent willingness to cooperate with the agency" as a salient criterion in the selection process. Certified caretakers are *expecting* agency monitoring, and at the very least are not negatively disposed toward such intervention.

The family care providers accommodate themselves to the outside evaluation of their performance and the subordination of parental discretion to the authority of an overseeing agency. They are able to do so by the partial substitution of the primary natural parenting analogy with a limited "occupational" one. In addition, by coping with evaluations and monitoring, mutually advantageous relationships with one's case worker tend to develop that eliminate the necessity of family care providers to "re-prove" themselves, provide intrinsic emotional satisfaction and gratification, and also serve as yardsticks against which to measure their performance in comparison to a population of "peers" with whom they seldom are in contact.

Conclusion

Family care providers, like all role incumbents, must function with some degree of role performance ambiguity and reconcile differing expectations from various role partners. The foster parent role is a particularly difficult position by virtue of its largely unspecified duties and ambiguous boundaries, internal inconsistencies among recognized role demands, and a minimum of anticipatory socialization and reference groups. In general, family care providers have attempted to handle these "role dilemmas," while simultaneously creating a personal role conception, by defining their role performance as more instrumental and therapeutic for the client than care by his or her natural parents, and as more effective and nurturing than the care an institution could ever provide.

In what direction might this role conceptualization take family care? There are a number of parallels with the literature on occupational ideologies, which deals with ways in which job holders define and consequently value their occupational positions. Many of these studies are about "helping" trades, professions, and occupations. While lowly ranked, these occupations are often viewed quite differently by those who fill them.

le performers stress their caring for others, a kind of sacred trust, in
rvice occupations. Similarly, we found that family care providers focus
e on important social values, such as caring for needy children, than on
less-lofty daily tasks required in the development of a professional
elf-image or ideology, consequently increasing their self-esteem and
occupational prestige and encouraging their continuation in the role.

To what extent are these role concepts of family care providers the
foundation for an occupational ideology? The results suggest that family
care providers would experience less role strain if they adhered to a strict
professional or occupational role definition. Indeed, this point of view seems
to underlie the independent suggestions of Alfred Kudushin and L. Davids
that the title "foster parent" be replaced with "child care worker." Such a
change would admittedly eliminate much of the ambiguity associated with
the role. Nevertheless, for family care providers for this population of
long-term, developmentally disabled placements, such an occupational role
definition would eliminate a great source of satisfaction—the intrinsic
pleasure to be derived from the relationship with the child. Further, an
exclusively professional or occupational role definition would lead to yet
another set of role strains. For example, it would accent an awareness of the
minimal anticipatory socialization and formal training received, highlight
the incompatibility of incumbents' being selected for the role on the basis of
such expressive criteria as one's child-rearing attitudes and relationship with
a spouse, and make the undeniable similarity between natural and foster
parent functions itself a source of role strain.

These directions cannot be determined without further study of the
multifaceted nature of foster parenting for various populations under the
guidance of different agencies. Further, any planned change toward
professionalization, such as by renaming the foster parent role, should be
based on anticipating the emergency of new sources of role strain as well as
on the need to eliminate old ones.

15
Future Research on Community Services

A knowledge of the social environment within which individuals learn, grow and participate, and to which they contribute is essential in planning a comprehensive community service network for people who are mentally retarded. The social environment is made up of the family, neighbors, friends, employers, service providers, and all the other ecological factors that impinge upon the individual.

Planning for the future cannot be based strictly on studying the past. Yet many issues suggested by previous research cry out for investigation. Because of the investment now being made in community systems, e.g., in buildings and in personnel, it is urgent that priority be given to the study of organizational and personal factors that make for uniformities and differences, for better or worse, in client outcomes. In its search for increased productivity, American industry has learned to look at systemwide conditions that encourage or discourage productive performances. Similar social research is needed in human services. In other words, cross-facility—agency differences in productivity (human outcomes)—need to be looked at with scientific objectivity. Methodologies are available for studying complex systems with many interacting variables: differentials in pay and working hours, supervisory styles, physical conditions (noise, color, or crowding) and psychological conditions (stress, autonomy, competition or motivation). All have a bearing on productivity, and can be translated into benefit/cost measures. Of course, it is necessary to have some consensus on what the "product" is and how it is to be measured and valued.

1. Personnel and Productivity. Given the cost of human service personnel, it is necessary to know if it makes a difference in productivity when changes in policy make it possible to attract and keep skilled personnel through competitive salary scales, including cost of living increments, with built-in opportunities for advancement. Another important and related issue is whether human service personnel can be expected to promote client development and independence if they are excluded from an involvement in the formation of treatment plans and little or no responsibility for client goal attainments.

2. *Effectiveness of Training Models.* There has been a long-term federal effort to redirect service specialists, psychologists, pediatricians, vocational rehabilitation counselors, and social workers, among others, in the provision of services to the mentally retarded. Federal funds in the last two decades were allocated to University Affiliated Facilities or programs associated with centers of higher education to encourage interdisciplinary training for professionals working with handicapped persons. In addition, substantial support to universities was accelerated in the 1970s under the federal mandate embodied in P.L. 94-142 and P.I.. 88-l64 for in-service training of personnel involved in the education of the handicapped. Data found in Chapter 8 show that the UAFs have, with relatively few federal dollars, produced a large number of graduates, yet little effort has been made to evaluate the impact of personnel with this special training on the quantity and quality of community services. We do know that some of those trained in federally supported programs have assumed leadership roles in the field. Whether their efforts and actions have made a critical difference remains to be investigated—if, indeed, it is possible to verify, given the external variables. Further, information on the extent to which generic service agencies actively provide treatment, evaluation, and other related tasks necessary for the development, protection, and support of the mentally retarded will also help us understand what special programs are required. While there are some obvious personnel shortages—say, for special educators, for occupational, physical, and speech therapists, and for qualified direct-care workers—there may be far less need for certain other professionals.

A critical issue, indeed, is the extent to which training efforts should be focused on making the generic practitioner more competent and confident in treating persons with a disability, and how much our resources should be focused on special training for persons who will have specialty careers in the field of mental retardation. One UAF (the University of Colorado), for example, has invested considerable time and talent in developing a replicable training package for collaborating personnel from other UAFs to provide training for primary physicians in private practice. An even more extensive effort was promoted by the American Academy of Pediatrics to educate pediatricians about their role in implementing P.L. 94-142. Unfortunately, there is limited evidence so far about the impact of these types of training efforts.

3. *Epidemiological Research.* Sound planning requires a knowledge of the developmental potentials presented by this population. Epidemiological data on community needs, service utilization data, and present staffing patterns need to be better understood. Demographic trends should be analyzed in greater detail. Considerable attention has already been given to the primary and secondary effects of changes in the age profile of our citizenry, say, in twenty or forty years, but relatively little attention has been

directed toward predictions of the future distribution of disability by age, type, degree, health status, educational need, or work potential.

4. *Residential Services.* Although several studies of the effects of "coming home" on the mentally retarded have been mounted in recent years, the findings reported in Chapter ll raise many unanswered questions. There is no agreement as to which measures of "benefit" should be used. Is the client more compliant, self-reliant, more skillful in staying out of jail, able to read better, keep a job, able to socialize, raise a family, or happier? No widely used inventory of social and adaptive skills indicates what is needed in different residential environments. A useful categorization of residential facilities and services would abandon terms such as "group home" or "community residence," which no longer convey meaningful information about program content and quality. The social environment for mentally retarded adults, for example, can vary according to the availability of (a) supportive human service networks, (b) future placements in more independent settings, and (c) number of candidates for open places. The extent to which the facilty is (d) integrated into the community, (e) the availability of vocational and recreational services, and (f) the extent to which residents have contact with family, friends, and neighbors in the community are also critical variables. Optimal staff training and staff-resident ratios remain to be determined as functions of, for example, (g) the degree of specialization of the facility, (h) the homogeneity of the population, (i) age, and (j) the objectives for individuals.

5. *Studies of Community Responses to Residential Integration.* Whether in a rural or urban location, community support and the existence of training options encourage adjustment to normalized living. Involvement of retarded citizens in the community is more a result of the social atmosphere than the density of the population.

The responses of most local communities to new residential facilities reflect their suspicion and fears, often leading to formal opposition, even when evidence is presented that property values will not be lowered nor neighborhoods disrupted. There is little consistency between the attitudes and actions of neighbors toward residential facilities and those who live in them. A neighborhood that appears agreeable to the location of a residence can turn against it, and opposition can subside once a facility is in place. Some researchers suggest that the more preparation that goes into readying a community, the more likely this will call attention to the presence of a residential facility, increasing the community opposition to its opening. Others hold the opposite view. Research is required to determine the conditions under which maximum community support can be obtained or, conversely, minimum perceived adverse impact.

6. *Early Intervention.* Most of the mild forms of mental retardation have no apparent physical cause and may be due to adverse environmental experience in early childhood. Despite the difficulty in ascertaining the etiology of mild mental retardation, this population can benefit enormously from behavioral research. For example, preliminary studies conducted by the Milwaukee Project identified forty women during pregnancy with

below-normal IQ scores from impoverished environments. After giving birth, mothers were randomly assigned to a control group receiving no special treatment or to an experimental group; the latter were given occupational, homemaking, and parenting training. Meanwhile, the infants of the mothers in the experimental group were provided over time with an intensive stimulation program, emphasizing achievement motivation, the development of problem-solving skills, and language acquisition. By school age the children reportedly had IQ scores averaging 26 points higher than those of the control group, and were far superior in verbal and numerical ability. Unfortunately, comprehensive followup studies have not been reported. A similar study in North Carolina called the Abecedarian Project also yielded positive results. Studies such as these, because of their social importance, deserve replication in other locations and under varying cultural and ecological conditions.

The importance of early intervention efforts is most evident in the oft-noted observation that community residences that teach self-care and home care skills are performing educational tasks that could be more appropriately taught at home when children are much younger. Underserved families need to be made aware that their mentally retarded children are capable of acquiring these skills, and that they are capable of managing behavior problems at early ages.

7. Education for Handicapped. Public Law 94-142 (Education for All Handicapped Children Act) represents one of the most important pieces of legislation for the handicapped ever passed, committing the United States to a "free appropriate public education" for all handicapped children. Yet there have been problems for administrators and teachers. Research is needed to assess the impact of its various provisions on children, their families, teachers, and school system.

The intent of P.L. 94-142 has been to promote the education of handicapped children in the least-restrictive environments, making it possible for handicapped children to learn in association with other children, and also for the latter to have the benefits of reciprocal effect. It is not clear if this policy, called "mainstreaming," has helped mentally retarded children to improve their intellectual performance. Some critics have suggested that the issue isn't where something is taught, but how well. Can all teachers learn to teach all handicapped children well, and if so, how best can they be trained to do so?

Much incidental learning occurs in an atmosphere devoted to academic excellence, one in which students are encouraged by the overall potential of the class to achieve academically. Jay Gottlieb, a psychologist who has studied attitude formation and the effects of mainstreaming (reported in Begab and Richardson 1975: 99-126) says that the relationship between proximity to the mentally retarded and attitudes toward them is uncertain and deserves further inquiry. He writes:

> The majority of evidence indicates that proximity is associated with increased rejection of mentally retarded individuals. The extent and nature of the contact, however, require explication. Information regarding the extent of

contact has been obtained in several ways, most often by asking the subject. The information is of limited value, however, since there is almost no way to corroborate the subject's statement. For example, when a subject indicates that he knew a retarded person, how can we be sure that the person he knew was actually retarded?

These misgivings are particularly critical in the field of education. The assumption is often made that placement in the same class promotes contact between handicapped and all other children. Yet it has also been noted that social isolation can take place without physical segregation.

Considerable evidence exists, in sum, that the causes of mental retardation are physical, biological, psychological, and social in origin, and often occur in combination in a single individual. Because of the frequent interaction of these elements in the development and behavior of children, knowledge must be gained from every branch of science.

To foster prevention and ameliorate the effects of mental retardation, the utilization of research findings needs to be increased. An effective and efficient information center at the national level, to identify and monitor current research related to the prevention of mental retardation, could serve this function. Future community services should be built on solid information and even more solid assessments of the conditions under which programs work.

16

Directions for the Future

Considerable progress has been made in the past twenty years in the development of community services. Not only have alternative residential arrangements been initiated, families have been tangibly assisted in the sometimes arduous task of keeping their retarded offspring at home. These changes have been accompanied by a gradual but perceptible increase in public acceptance of handicapped and mentally retarded individuals as citizens who are entitled to lead lives as normal as possible. There is an increasing appreciation of the fact that mentally retarded people, just as other citizens, have a right to human dignity.

Despite the considerable progress of the past twenty years, there is still a need to improve and integrate federally supported efforts, as well as to increase coordination between federal, state, and local agencies to achieve a comprehensive approach defining service, research, and training needs. The problems are complex, dynamic, and intricately interlocked with the fabric of society at large and particularly with its more disadvantaged segments. What is best, and for whom? Who can do it, at what cost, where and how? To these questions there are only partial or fragmented answers.

The advances in delivery of community services, although a revolution in one sense, has actually been a gradual process that has accelerated in recent years. The progress made thus far has not resulted in a massive movement of mentally retarded people from the back wards to the back streets. Some abuses and some problems remain, since no movement of this magnitude can be carried forward without misstep or error.

Current Research

Scattered but systematically collected evidence has given us some indications of how to avoid recreating mini-institutions in the community. Research on the failings of large institutions stresses not only the size of the facilities, but the monocratic nature of the decision-making processes, which excludes both employees and residents. Inappropriate environments range from the overly protective to the downright neglectful, with depersonalization and social isolation prevailing.

Although few followup studies are available, the past research on success in community placement has focused on the following factors: the type of maladaptive behavior residents manifest before and during placement; the personal and vocational skills developed; the progress in development of satisfactory interpersonal relationships; the environmental variables, including size and physical accommodations as influences on behavior; the attitudes of staff and their participation in decision-making; the homogeneity or heterogeneity of the population; and the degree of program structure and its quality.

Thus far research results are suggestive but not absolutely convincing in determining what makes a community residence effective and for whom or, conversely, what leads to failure in helping a retarded person with this or that characteristic. The data have suggested the benefits of smallness but are not fully conclusive. By and large, staff attitudes and training are among the more critical factors affecting client growth. Nonetheless, the smaller units have a greater potential for success, inasmuch as morale and decentralized decision-making are more easily fostered. Bringing more caretakers into units and increasing investment in more labor did not of itself improve the adaptive behavior of retarded adults. Rather, special skills training has been beneficial. Striking differences in programs are found to be based on staff values, operating procedures, and the quality of the living environment. It is interesting that client behaviors in the larger residential settings have had little direct relationship to the cost of care. Currently, there are no useful measures to determine objectively why some programs succeed despite their being less costly.

ISSUES

To judge from the available research, there are apparent advantages in having a variety of community residences to meet the varying needs of persons of different ages, skills, temperament, and impairment. They may cover a wide range in size; varying combinations of staff and staff/client ratios may be applicable in different situations. Therefore, if better community residential care is to be offered,

- greater emphasis should be placed on the training of management techniques,
- direct-care staff should participate in decision-making, and
- clients' preexisting social relationships and social networks must be considered during movement from one setting to another.

Federal and state guidelines for residential programs should minimize unnecessary and arbitrary restrictions on both staff and clients, particularly those that limit program creativity and flexiblity. A quality of living should be encouraged to support or permit the fulfillment of personal preferences, views, and capabilities. It is also apparent that more well controlled, longitudinal, multidimensional studies are required to assess the impact of combinations of environmental and programmatic factors on the mentally retarded in community residential settings.

Community Service Systems

Future services must be people-oriented, remaining accountable but flexibly operated, with a coherent goal-directed philosophy. No single simple set of solutions exists to the problems of successful service delivery, nor is there any formula to avoid competition for finite resources among divergent groups within the human services delivery spectrum. But certain basic principles can be extracted, focusing on what is needed to evolve a national policy based on a respect for human dignity, and consistent with those national values that characterize our society.

With the tremendous growth in delivery of community services, compounded by the deinstitutionalization efforts, progress in achieving a coordinated service system has been impeded by the complexity of funding mechanisms, bureaucratic restrictions, poor coordination, and difficulty in adjustment of some persons who have been relocated from a restricted setting into the open community. Increased demands for time-consuming paperwork for managers to assure accountability have slowed the trend toward greater interdependence of systems of services, including the generic service systems.

The systems are complex, and participation in them generates concern about issues of extent of control, rights of clients, ownership of facilities or programs, and the related funding streams that support them. Furthermore, the systems have a background of jurisdictional disputes and inherent adversarial relationships.

The mental retardation/developmental disablity system is best considered in the context of the larger system within which it operates. As a schema, it presents a very complicated array or distribution of services, having a multitude of components with interfaces that often seem unworkable. Yet this very complexity is normal; what is needed is some additional ingredient to support the person who has less capacity to cope, less "street wisdom."

Part of the problem relates to the shock of transition from a closed system (institutionally oriented) to an open system with uncertain boundaries. It is more difficult to achieve systemwide objectives under these conditions. On local, state, and national levels, many planning efforts have been spawned and demonstrations mounted, but the results are limited to idiosyncratic successes, dependent on extraordinary local leadership, commitment, creativity, and unusual community receptivity.

Providing a comprehensive array of services for a continuum of care, given the network of entitlement programs, is a complex problem. Current planning has been dominated by the issue of deinstitutionalization without sufficient concern for the development of a broad-based alternative system for those in need. Assistance for the severely handicapped can be enabling when such care is goal-oriented or actively therapeutic and restorative, rather than merely directed to sustaining life.

There is need to try diverse approaches; no single formula to assure effective services currently exists. "Macro" solutions do not necessarily apply to "micro" needs in small communities. The need is not to revolutionize the system totally, but to modify it. As one participant in a recent conference put it, this is no easy task, because "if you don't think that we have a system, try to change that system." Some ambiguity will always exist, but what is favorable must be used, built on what has been learned, while modifying or eliminating only inefficient, wasteful, and ineffective elements.

Waste can be reduced by guaranteeing access to generic services for all groups, including the mentally retarded, while dealing with the unique needs of this population. To do this, the overall national demographics that reflect a decrease in child population and an increase in our aged population must be considered. Furthermore, the baby boom has now reached young adulthood with its share of impaired members. These trends affect the plans for future services and those for whom they must be designed.

Specific program areas, now almost universally deficient, must be bolstered. These include work-oriented training for the severely retarded, access to mental health services, satisfactory case management services, and the availability of physical rehabilitation programs and care by other medical specialists. These deficiencies are all cited as causes of failure in community placement of deinstitutionalized clients. Unless community service models can be demonstrated to be comprehensive and effective, they may become an endangered species with less than unanimous support from parents, professionals, labor unions, and fiscal experts.

RECOMMENDATIONS

Community care is best based on four key principles that determine the quality of life: *normalization, the developmental model, individualization, and self-actualization.* A successful system offering humane and comprehensive community care must strive to achieve the following goals:

- Integration of generic services into a client-oriented system.
- Insurance that the system responds to human needs rather than bureaucratic rules.
- Promotion of individual growth and development to the maximum degree possible.
- Provision for freedom of choice from among available options for clients and their families.
- Encouragement of the use of a competitive model so there is an opportunity for participation in service delivery by private, proprietary, and voluntary nonprofit sectors as well as public agencies, both generic and specialized.

- Promotion of natural arrangements whereby people can take more responsibility for one another in self-reliant communities.
- Maximization of productivity in line with the changing economic picture and the increasing cost of energy, housing, and transportation, such as having clients care for themselves, transport themselves, and receive training so they can produce goods and services and receive adequate pay.
- Development of consortia of providers to improve service coordination.
- Expectation that most generic services, including education, vocational training, work, or day activity programs, occur away from the place of the residence.
- Reshaping of the role of traditional institutions, if retained, with an emphasis on intensive short-term treatment and crisis intervention.
- Fostering of continuity of services and provision for the constancy in caretaking so essential to assuring the personal growth, social and vocational competence of impaired persons.
- Stimulation of the development of community care through clear and consistent federal regulations.
- Full participation for mentally retarded persons in the life in their communities and the opportunity to share its responsibilities.
- Assurance of opportunities that mentally retarded persons may make their own decisions and direct their own lives to the greatest extent possible.
- Guarantees that those who are among the multitudes of Americans who require assistance in communication through nonverbal means or through augmentative communication techniques receive this training, to promote their integration into the community.
- Provision of an array of needed services in all communities.
- Decentralization and distribution of services on a regional or geographic basis, emphasizing the use of trained indigenous personnel.
- Development of service delivery models with unique characteristics that will work in differing environments. This approach recognizes that there is no one community, but many types of communities and subdivisions with unique characteristics and differences, and that these should be dealt with in their own way. Long-term trends indicate a continuing redistribution, including urbanization, of our population. There is a now a new migration to rural areas where there are traditions of self-sufficiency.
- Support of the role of the family, whether natural or foster, and recognition of the growing tendency of parents to maintain and care for their retarded offspring at home so that stress should increasingly be placed on respite services for parents and home-based health care, as well as training activities, particulary for young infants and preschool children. (Examples include the use of itinerant teachers, video casette instructional materials, interactive cable TV systems and, as reported earlier, more modern telecommunication techniques.)

- Maintenance and improvement of efficacy of the public schools, to assure that each child will receive a free and appropriate education that recognizes individuality, worth, and potential.

Educational Services

Substantial evidence indicates that P.L. 94-142 (Education for All Handicapped Children Act) has produced considerable progress in achieving free appropriate public education for handicapped children. A 1984 report from the U.S. Department of Education of the 1982–83 school year census indicates that 4,298,327 children are now receiving public educational services, an increase of 589,739 children since the first careful child count was conducted in 1976–77.

Under the current legislation, states are mandated to establish "child find" programs, to locate, identify, and evaluate all eligible handicapped children, to thereafter conduct nondiscriminatory evaluations, and to place children in the least-restrictive environment consistent with their special needs. The legislation also assures parents of the guarantee of due process, including the right to an impartial hearing to assure that the child's rights are protected, whether in private or public educational facilities. Providers are required to offer relevant in-service training to the staff and to assure the provision of "related services," including psychological services, social services, medical assessment, and required therapies (speech, physical, and occupational). The overall objective of these measures is to provide individualized instruction based on the child's needs and to assure that related services necessary to support instructional activities are provided.

OBJECTIVES

Although some programs meet the educational needs of handicapped children they serve, current legislation and its implementation have not fully ensured this, insofar as large numbers of eligible children do not yet receive individualized teaching and related services. Implementation of P.L. 94-142 needs to remain a high priority, with emphasis on the following:

- Reaching all children eligible for services by expanding outreach efforts and coordinating the activities of early identification with the medical services delivery system.
- Assuring education for all eligible children so no individual or group of children is given preference or denied services by degree of handicap.
- Developing individual approaches to assure that health services and related therapies are coordinated and integrated with the educational programs.
- Assuring continuation and improvement of federal support for personnel preparation in the fields of special education, pediatrics,

neurology, psychology, child development, and vocational rehabilitation. Special attention should be given to in-service training activities, with an emphasis on interdisciplinary training of educational and related services personnel.

- Expanding federal and state monitoring and technical assistance to ensure full compliance with the law, including efforts to "mainstream" children, wherever feasible, and to provide specialized educational programs to children with special needs.

PRESCHOOL PROGRAMS

An increasing body of research-based knowledge supports the view that early intervention, beginning shortly after birth, can be effective with many handicapped infants and toddlers, including those recognized as retarded. Better language capability in later years, for example, has its foundations in this period.

While P.L. 94-142 encourages states, through small fiscal incentives, to offer education for children three to five years of age, the option to provide these services is clearly left to the states. As a result, the growth in reported services for children in this age bracket has been slow. However, preschool special programs for the mentally retarded and developmentally disabled population predominantly have been supported by state or local mental health/mental retardation agencies or by grants from the federal Office of Special Education's Handicapped Children's Early Education Program (HCEEP). Handicapped children have also been integrated into the Head Start programs in response to the mandate that such programs must include at least 10 percent handicapped children.

RECOMMENDATIONS

Early intervention and education measures are essential to minimize or mitigate the adverse impacts of handicapping conditions on children and their families. The federal government, in concert with state educational authorities, needs to develop a systematic plan to encourage and assist states and localities to expand preschool education. The plan should include the following provisions:

- Provide fiscal incentives for expansion of early identification and intervention efforts.
- Establish close working relationships between the medical and educational communities to coordinate followup of high risk infants, to provide for the early identification of disabilities and to offer early intervention services.
- Integrate required "related services" into the educationally oriented intervention efforts.
- Emphasize assistance to the family to help them understand the needs of their handicapped child and to help foster the carry-over of

instruction from school or center-based intervention programs to the home. This includes offering home-start or home-based intervention services as options, particularly in rural areas where transportation is not readily available.

- Provide technical assistance to agencies to enhance intergovernmental cooperation, using such models as the American Association of University Affiliated Programs'–sponsored "Interagency Collaborative Project to Improve Services to Preschool Handicapped Children."

Financing Services

It has been said that program people propose, but budget people dispose. In the face of increasing competition for scarce resources, economic issues remain a critical component of planning for future community services. Unfortunately, the delivery of human services, including those to mentally retarded individuals and their families, is fragmented, and a fixation on funding streams has produced inconsistent policies. Many experts feel that human service agencies must decrease their dependency on government programs, eliminate components of the burgeoning bureaucracy, and heed the backlash against supporting special groups.

More than 1.7 million mentally retarded Americans now receive some form of public income maintenance for medical, educational, social, or residential support. Many of the estimated 230,000 in long-term large residential facilities, including nursing homes (100,000), state institutions for mentally ill (12,000) and for the mentally retarded (118,000), should or could be in community-based active treatment programs or living facilities. The total federal support, including Titles XIX and XX, vocational rehabilitation, developmental disabilities, and educational entitlement of special targeted programs was, in 1983, more than $7.5 billion. This was 49% of a nationwide program estimated at $15.3 billion. In the 1982 expenditures for various types of residential care recently reported by Bruininks from the Center for Residential and Community Services at the University of Minnesota, the average daily cost of care per affected person in a group community residence was $42.77 (or $15,600 per year), living at home or in foster care costs $16 per person (or $6,800 per year). This compares with $86.25 per day and more than $31,000 annually per client for institutional care. If the current patterns of expenditures and inflation continue, it is projected that by 1986 the overall costs of the MR/DD system will reach more than twice the 1980 level, and one-third higher than the 1983 level of expenditure.

In view of the discrepancy in cost between community care and institutional care, a new strategy needs to be developed to maximize the use of cost effective services supported by federal and local funds. The emphasis for those clients who require structured programs would be on active treatment, rehabilitation, and avoidance of inappropriate institutionalization. This strategy would provide for the kind of income and service structure that would support independent living, productivity, normalization, and life in the least-restrictive environment for as many mentally retarded individuals as possible. Supporting families to manage their progeny at home, rather than providing unintended but real fiscal incentives to institutionalize relatives, is cost-effective. (It could also help ease the family's psychosocial stress.)

It will require changes by governmental agencies at all levels to reallocate current resources and the use of any new resources and creative financing techniques as catalysts to alter the system and develop new service approaches.

RECOMMENDATIONS

A strategy for change in the funding of services for the disabled must be multidimensional and multidisciplinary. It will require a new management approach, flexible policies, and creative, joint state and federal collaboration in financing and programming. It cannot be forced by creating unrealistic time frames to reduce or eliminate the institutional system.

The Health Care Financing Administration (HCFA) has the largest single responsibility in financing residential care. It may be possible to make changes in the way HCFA operates within the current law; regulations as they now exist require only minor changes. The financing of services could be organized to promote continuity of care around homogeneous target groups, such as the mentally retarded and developmentally disabled, the aged and mentally ill. Each of these groups could become part of a long-term care initiative that would permit the federal government to deal simultaneously with special groups but preserve their ability to deal with special needs, such as those of the mentally retarded. This approach could force the federal, state, and local agencies into a format of total program budgeting. In this, states will have to consider their need for a spectrum of residential and community services: i.e., for the most-economical alternatives. This change would also require the development and implementation of a system of case management, program accountability, and the necessary support services.

To develop the continuum of care system for the retarded and developmentaly disabled, the following are necessary:

- Incentives to move toward less costly and more appropriate residential placement alternatives, including realistic family support for home care.
- A more flexible reimbursement based on levels of required care and services.
- Data on costs, client movement, and flow of persons into different parts of the service delivery system while protecting confidentiality. Under such a system, more normalized levels of care should cost less but be no less attractive, profitable, or easy to finance.

- Funding of active treatment, where required, by individual need under Title XIX, both for residential programs and nonresidential day programs.
- Encouragement of deinstitutionalization efforts and institutional phase-down with tighty monitored utilization review and rate setting policies, and fiscal incentives for conversion of funds for use in normalizing community programs.
- Discouragement by the federal government of further institutional investments in capital construction which, after completion, tends to lock in reimbursement for institutional care for a certain number of beds at the apparent expense of community care options.

New initiatives are needed to support these preferences both in program, theory, regulation, and law. An increase in local innovation and control is desirable, with consumer choice and technical assistance provided by federally supported research, training, and program development agencies.

In summary, the system of financing services must be based on proper management; it should make use of budgetary incentives to shift resources into community care. It should be program-oriented, support normalization, foster the development of less-expensive noninstitutional options, and be fiscally attractive to state and local governments. It should not merely pay for someone living in a residential bed, but help finance services for individuals or groups of needy citizens wherever they reside.

Management and Accountability

It is possible to reduce the difficulties found in being in compliance with various laws and administrative regulations. The growth of federal programs for the mentally retarded, accompanied by specific regulations and guidelines, has no doubt increased the quantity and quality of services over the past decade. Yet it has been accompanied by a tendency toward centralized decision-making and an increase in paperwork and unnecessary jurisdictional rigidity. It has raised serious questions in the minds of both consumers and advocates as to whom the system is accountable. Is it to federal, state, or local governments?

What is often overlooked is that ultimate accountability is to the consumer and his or her family or representative. Viewed from this perspective, it is evident that in the name of accountability the client's freedom of movement, freedom of choice, and what Perske has called "dignity of risk" are constantly at risk. There is a strong tendency for managers to want to deal with numbers and put groups in boxes on charts, rather than to deal with an individual's programmatic needs.

The current trend places a special stress on fiscal accountability and eligibility for benefits. Mistakenly, however, the quality of the service is equated with performance by employees. Efforts are made to relate gains in client functioning to employee performance. While fiscal accountability is absolutely necessary, a plea must be made for flexibility in funding it, so long as it is used in an entirely legal manner.

Eligibility for benefits based on disability and on economic need remains a more thorny issue. There has never been any significant evidence of malingering in the mental retardation and developmental disability fields. A difficult question remains concerning the dubious and arbitrary exclusion of many who are only marginally able citizens. It has often been observed that SSI eligibility standards vary from office to office, not so much on economic grounds as on the degree of retardation or developmental disability. Other examples of arbitrariness are found in the disincentives for work built into the SSI and SSDI programs.

Paperwork demands have mushroomed as a result of increased regulations and concerns about productivity. Workers now have less time to spend with clients. Employee training is still inadequate. Client gains may clearly be related to social, physical, environmental, or programmatic factors well beyond the control of individual employees. Who is responsible for client improvements, and how are we to measure employee performance under these circumstances?

What we have seen in the 1970s has been the operationalizing of the ideology of the 1960s. The 1980s offer us an opportunity to determine what works and why, and to try to make the whole complex system work better. This will not be accomplished if unrealistic demands for data (paper accountability) or punitive threats are made against employees. We need to develop both process and outcome measures, reasonable information systems that offer feedback to the person providing the data input, the true "consumers" of the data system.

We must facilitate mechanisms for habilitation planning, case management, client tracking, program planning, and budgeting. Clearly, information systems must be parsimonious in the use of resources, relevant to client and management needs, and designed to adapt to this period of technological change. Evaluation systems must be educationally useful to those being evaluated but flexible enough to deal with the cultural differences in our client populations and to rationalize those standards that lead to creative programmatic approaches.

RECOMMENDATIONS

Because of the proliferation of data collection systems which are not directed to improving the quality of life for clients, there is a need to avoid overzealous attempts at useless data gathering. Systems must be developed that are clearly user friendly and have both value to the persons providing the input and offer useful information for those studying the resultant data that is produced. Management flexibility must be encouraged, while maintaining high standards for programs. Regulations must not be oppressive, nor should evaluation systems be insensitive to human needs. Management and accountability can be made more effective and efficient if the following suggestions are followed:

- Utilize two way information systems to provide not only data about clients, but feedback to providers about client movement and program effectiveness.
- Guarantee confidentiality about clients and their families in the use of any information system.
- Allow for sufficient flexibility and autonomy for staff so they may pursue goals in the interests of clients while at the same time ensuring fiscal accountability.
- Avoid bureaucratic stultification that accompanies centralization of responsibility and authority.
- Utilize less intrusive techniques not merely based on hypothetical levels of care. The instruments must reflect the needs of individual clients and of the community.
- Establish a standardized mechanism for reporting client abuse and neglect.
- Develop better techniques for establishing priorities between institutional and community-based programs, and for supporting families who choose to care for their retarded relatives at home.
- Stimulate staff productivity by humanizing the work environment, improving promotional opportunities in career ladder structures, fostering staff commitment, and encouraging and rewarding ingenuity, creativity, and productivity.
- Provide a continuum of service for all clients. If the marketplace alone determines what service will be provided, there will be serious gaps in services, especially those needed by "difficult" or unattractive clients (older, less responsive, facially disfigured, deformed, or inarticulate).
- Provide sufficient incentives to encourage small service providers who offer diversity and program alternatives.
- Be open to new ideas and new solutions. At the same time, encourage the collection of a reliable data base to support the formulation of future policy decisions.

Advocacy, Rights, and Full Citizenship

The right of all citizens to full participation in community life and societal membership, up to their capacities, is a basic tenet of the community mental retardation and developmental disability movement. The right to an appropriate community placement is a fundamental one.

Until the past decade the legal profession had only limited interest in mental retardation. This has rapidly changed with an increasing supply of interested and trained lawyers, especially through the activities of the protection and advocacy systems and legal aid offices. In part, as a result of earlier litigation, legislative advances, and mounting public awareness of long-established rights, the need and demand for formal and informal advocates have expanded exponentially. Another substantial change is represented by the growth of the self-advocacy movement and the increasing demands by retarded persons for a role in decision-making.

Many problems are still unsolved, including assurance of appropriate due process mechanisms for both institutionalized and community care clients, access to appropriate public education, appropriate handling of the mentally retarded offenders (allegedly characterized by many examples of "assembly line injustice") and, finally, provision of sophisticated guardianship or alternative services tailored to fit the individual's unique needs and capacities. What must be assured is the right to a good start in life, the right to access for the needed services, and the right to a normal physical environment and a normal pattern of living, preferably at home or in smaller community-based facilities.

RECOMMENDATIONS

Informal settlement processes are required to solve problems at the local and state levels. In the face of a growing tendency toward litigation and difficulties in enforcing any resultant court judgments and decrees, it appears that individual rights of the retarded would be more effectively guaranteed if legal efforts focused on developing on-site administrative mechanisms and a spectrum of oversight resources, such as human rights committees, ombudsmen, and grievance procedures. This will mean that additional trained independent advocates will be needed to provide representation and to work on pragmatic problem-solving to assure individual rights and, particularly, access to required services. This could be the major future direction of protection and advocacy systems, along with attempting to identify areas of client abuse, utilizing both child and adult protective services.

Since all people should have a chance to learn their rights and responsibilities and to receive training on how to advocate, the self-advocacy movement should be encouraged and supported, with training begun in early adolescence and particular effort made to prepare individuals to represent themselves as advisors to decision-making bodies. Self-advocacy and protection of rights need to be buttressed by:

- Vigorous action by state government to safeguard the legal and human rights of all disabled persons.
- Preservation of existing statutory rights, such as the rights to nondiscriminatory treatment.
- State-run programs to train independent advocates who will provide representation and other pragmatic problem-solving approaches to assure individual rights.
- Development of a broad spectrum of oversight and dispute settlement mechanisms, including but not limited to human rights committees, ombudsmen, and impartial grievance mechanisms.
- Initiation of specific projects to deal with retarded and disabled offenders, including ways of guarding their rights, encouraging

appropriate handling of the criminal process for those who are partially competent, providing treatment programs that focus on requirements dictated by the disability and not merely the resultant behavior that brought the individual to the attention of the legal authorities, and establishing satisfactory due process safeguards to assure appropriate residential and educational placements.

- Equal access to housing opportunities through such means as elimination of exclusionary zoning laws to permit the operation of group residences in typical residential neighborhoods, and setting aside a percentage of new accommodations for mentally retarded and handicapped people in all federally supported housing.

Vocational Training

Self-advocates are dismayed that the mentally retarded are offered only menial or degrading jobs when seeking employment. Part of the problem stems from inadequate job preparation or training, and part from outright discrimination. Tested and documented training curricula, however, have been developed in the past decade to teach even the severely retarded to carry out complex vocationally oriented tasks.

Instead of being productive citizens, many retarded adults are still being maintained unnecessarily in a dependent state. Documentation supports the claim that dollars invested in vocational training yield a manyfold increase in income from productive work on the part of the mentally retarded.

RECOMMENDATIONS

At the federal, state, and local levels, incentives should be provided to foster the development and utilization of training methods to improve skills and abilities and, thereby, enhance employment potential. The following measures would be useful in dealing with the problem:

- Dissemination of improved methods—a wide distribution of program information to providers.
- An educational effort aimed at potential industrial employers to inform them of the skills, potential, and positive qualities of mentally retarded workers.
- Provision, wherever possible, of competitive employment for the mentally retarded and developmentally disabled. The next best option is a means of subsidized employment with fiscal incentives for the employer. The final option is the sheltered workshop.

It is essential that the productivity potential of the mentally retarded be utilized. This is both the most humane and cost-effective approach that can be promoted.

Labor Issues

The quality of life for the mentally retarded depends on the quality of people working in residential settings and nonresidential service programs. Thus far, no one has satisfactorily defined the optimum level of specialized training required to care for retarded persons on a day-to-day basis or what formal credentials may be necessary. The evidence is that interdisciplinary training, as well as on-the-job training, can be a useful approach in the hands of competent trainers.

The problems that now exist in the labor area include the displacement of public employees from institutional positions, the growth of services provided by profit-making or nonprofit voluntary agency vendors, the lack of a reasonable hierarchy of job opportunities for direct-care staff compounded by poor pay scales, and the blurring of professional roles in interdisciplinary settings, with their increased emphasis on team-directed habilitation or education as the active treatment modality.

RECOMMENDATIONS

Attention must be paid to the retraining and relocation of current institutional employees for community roles concomitant with the phasedown of institutions. Interdisciplinary and on-the-job training procedures are required along with the following measures:

- Use of reasonable career ladders with fiscal incentives for the industrious, productive, and responsible employees.
- Stress on professional training and role performance in new community-based service networks, including the development of improved supervisory or administrative skills and mechanisms to assist workers from ethnic and social minorities. (As services are distributed in a more geographically disbursed pattern, ethnically indigenous personnel should be employed where possible. This policy enhances outreach efforts and improves community relations.)
- Rewards for employees who are committed and creative in their jobs, since these characteristics have the best chance of making community services or, for that matter, all services work more effectively.

Role of Developmental Disability Councils

Excessive regulatory procedures and undefined roles with regard to state service delivery systems have hampered Developmental Disability Councils in their operations. Yet they have a potentially important role to play in providing consumer input into state planning efforts. They are a useful vehicle for bringing consumers together with state and local agency policy-makers in various departments serving the mentally retarded and developmentally disabled population.

RECOMMENDATIONS

The continuation of the Developmental Disability Councils with further clarification of their planning and advisory roles in their respective states is desirable. These councils should advise state agencies on the evaluation of programs, but not be the principal agent responsible for conducting evaluations. At their discretion, DD Councils, should utilize funds to support innovative programs, and to provide technical assistance activities for state, local, and voluntary agencies in delivery of community services.

- DD Council members should play an important role as intermediaries between governmental officials and public and consumer groups. In that role, they can educate the public and interpret policy issues.

Future Research

Considerable research has centered on the areas of program efficacy and on prevention strategies. Exciting progress has been made in biological research in the neurosciences, and the future undoubtedly holds considerable opportunities for enhancing our knowledge about to the causes of mental retardation. Future research efforts should lead to increases in prevention and offer new opportunities for treatment—how best to deliver services in a more effective way.

GOALS

The relatively minute amount of resources expended on research in mental retardation and developmental disabilities (particularly as compared to the huge expenditure on service activities) clearly justifies an increased investment in research activities. Such research efforts should be expanded in both biological and behavioral areas including:

- Research emphasizing prevention that will point to new directions for community-based prevention efforts. (Research on the application of the new technologies was noted in Chapter 6.)
- Organizational research on service delivery, including studies of the impact of size, programmatic approaches, environmental circumstances, and medications on the behavior of clients. Studies are also needed to examine the impact on the family of maintaining retarded relatives at home, or of providing family supports and respite services and of utilizing the family as therapists for their own child.
- Research on the most useful techniques for early identification and intervention.
- Research on attitudinal changes toward the handicapped, the impact

of deinstitutionalization, and the effect of the media on this process. More studies of the effects of mainstreaming in the public education system are also needed.

- Research on structural changes in the delivery system, including the roles of private, voluntary, or public service providers. These would include the impact of contracts for services and the organizational approaches to coordinating services. Better prevalence data from new epidemiological studies would assist such investigations.

Studies are needed to define the changing role of professionals and other treatment personnel in evolving decentralized service delivery models. The issues of the effectiveness of staff training procedures and the best methods for increasing staff productivity have to be investigated. How do staff members interact with one another? With clients? With members of the community? In summary, we need to determine what helps the retarded and what does not. We also need better tools to determine who will succeed in community placement and to assess the critical factors in successful community living environments.

Prevention

Prevention will always remain a key element in an enhanced effort for comprehensive community services. There has been only limited progress in the implementation of prevention, despite advances in knowledge of the effectiveness of both biological and environmental prevention measures.

GOALS

Efforts to prevent mental retardation and developmental disabilities must include:

- Expansion of biological prevention efforts stressing the most cost-effective elements, including genetic counseling services and prevention of exposure of pregnant women to toxic substances and to occupational hazards.
- Expansion of efforts to (a) prevent fetal alcoholism syndrome, (b) improve prenatal care with regional perinatal care networks for those with high-risk of adverse perinatal outcome, (c) decrease drug usage during pregnancy that has potentially adverse effects on the fetus and neonate, and (d) continue public assistance to nutritionally at-risk mothers.
- Expansion of regionalized perinatal care with research on how to improve technology in intensive care for the high-risk neonates.
- Expansion of statewide and regional programs for metabolic screening of all newborns to detect and treat all infants having metabolic disorders.
- Expansion and improvement in the followup of high-risk infants,

including assistance in early identification, coupled with application of improved early intervention methods.

- Reduction of preventable postnatally acquired mental retardation. These causes include trauma due to accidents and poisonings with household substances and drugs, infectious diseases that are preventable through immunizations, and toxic exposures to substances such as lead found in the paint and plaster in old buildings, and in industrial settings.
- Elimination or reduction of those conditions of poverty and social disadvantage which frequently lead to mild retardation.

Reports from Sweden indicate that mild mental retardation can be reduced by a combination of medical, social service, and educational efforts. Considering the cost to the American society of caring for relatively dependent or unproductive citizens with mental retardation and severe developmental disabilities, we should provide further incentives to expand prevention efforts in the future and motivate governmental agencies to assure that all citizens have access to such services. This effort can be accomplished by improving the capacity of state and local agencies to provide the aforementioned services. Expertise and resources are available to achieve this goal at University Affiliated Facilities and Mental Retardation Research Centers, and from the Federal Office of Special Education (Department of Education) and Division of Maternal and Child Health (Department of Health and Human Services).

Looking to the Future

The movement to repatriate the mentally retarded citizens of the United States and offer them full citizenship and legal rights can be viewed as an inevitable consequence of our continuing evolution as a democratic society. Concomitant with the achievement of full citizenship is the right to live where one chooses, in a manner comparable to other citizens. Therefore, the justifiable trend toward community care for almost all the retarded and handicapped, with the possible exception of the most medically dependent population, seems likely to continue. Along these lines, there should be a continued search for improved prevention measures, for better ways to provide services, and for methods to promote increased educational and social skills among the retarded.

From moral, ethical, and economic standpoints, it is in everyone's interest to foster the development of community services and maintain steady progress toward this goal. In doing so, mentally retarded and developmentally disabled people will have the greatest possible opportunity to move from dependency to becoming useful participants and contributers to our society.

References

Allard, Mary Ann, and Gail E. Toff. 1980.
  Current and Future Development of Intermediate Care Facilities for the Mentally Retarded: A Study of State Officials. Washington, D.C.: Human Services Research Institute.
Ambinder, W., et al. 1962.
  "Role phenomena and foster care for disturbed children."*American Journal of Orthopsychiatry* 32: 32–39.
Bada, Henrietta S., and Charles W. Fitch. 1983.
  "Use of transcutaneous doppler ultrasound techniques in newborn infants." *Perinatology-Neonatology* 7: 27–35.
Baroff, George. 1980.
  "On 'Size' and the quality of residential care: A second look." *Mental Retardation* 18:113–18.
Begab, Michael J., and Stephen A. Richardson. 1975.
  The Mentally Retarded and Society: A Social Science Perspective. Baltimore, London, and Tokyo: University Park Press.
Bellamy, G. Thomas, Martin R. Sheehan, Robert H. Horner, and Shawn M. Boles. 1980.
  Community Programs for Severely Handicapped Adults: An Analysis of Vocational Opportunities. Eugene: University of Oregon Center on Human Development. Mimeo.
Bennett, Marianne, James F. Budde, and Elinor Gollay. (N.d.)
  Consumers on the move: The Developmental Disabilities self-help advocacy movement.
Benson, Philip P. 1971.
  The Biochemistry of Development. Clinics in Developmental Medicine No. 37. Spastics International Medical Publishers, London: Wm. Heinemann Med. Publishers, and J.B. Lippincott, Philadelphia.
Bergman, J.S.. 1975.
  Community Homes for the Retarded. Lexington, Mass.: D.C. Heath.
Berkson, Gerson, and Daniel Romer. 1980a.
  "Social ecology of supervised communal facilities for mentally disabled adults." *American Journal of Mental Deficiency* 85:219–28.
  1980b. "Predictors of affiliation." *American Journal of Mental Deficiency* 85:229–42.

1980c. "Predictors of social choice." *American Journal of Mental Deficiency* 85:243–52.

Birenbaum, Arnold. 1970.
"On managing a courtesy stigma." *Journal of Health and Social Behavior* 11: 196–206.

Birenbaum, Arnold, and M.B. Ahmed. 1978.
"Recruitment, training and utilization of community mental health workers." *Sociological Symposium* 23: 122–34.

Birenbaum, Arnold, and M.A. Re. 1980.
"Finding and keeping family care providers." Pp. 104-20 in Herbert Cohen and David Kligler, eds., *Urban Community Care for the Developmentally Disabled.* Springfield, Ill.: Charles Thomas.

Birenbaum, Arnold, and Samuel Seiffer. 1976.
Resettling Retarded Adults in a Managed Community. New York: Praeger.

Blatt, Burton. 1966.
Christmas in Purgatory: A Photographic Essay. Boston: Allyn and Bacon.

Bradley, Valerie J. 1980.
Mental Disabilities Services in the 80's: Maintenance of Public Accountability in a Privately Operated System.

Breen, Paula, and Gary Richman. 1979.
"Evaluation of the developmental disability concept." Pp 3–6 in Ronald Wiegerink and John N. Pelosi, eds., *Developmental Disabilities: The DD Movement.* Baltimore: Paul N. Brookes.

Brownell, Gordon L., Thomas F. Budinger, Paul C. Lautenburg and Patrick L. McGeer. 1982.
"Positron tomography and nuclear magnetic resonance imaging." *Science* 215: 619–26.

Bruininks, Robert H., Mary J. Kudla, Colleen A. Wieck, and Florence A. Hauber. 1980.
"Management problems in community residential facilities." *Mental Retardation* 18:125–29.

Bruininks, Robert H., et al. 1983.
The 1982 National Census of Residential Facilities: Summary Report. Minneapolis: University of Minnesota Center for Residential and Community Services.

Cantor, M.D. 1975.
The formal and informal social support systems of older New Yorkers. A paper presented at the 10th annual International Congress of Gerontology, Jerusalem, 25 June 1975.

Child Welfare League of America. 1962.
Quantitative Approaches to Parent Selection. New York: Child Welfare League of America. Mimeo.

Cohen, Herbert J., and David Kligler, eds. 1980.
Urban Community Care for the Developmentally Disabled. Springfield: Charles C. Thomas, Publisher.

Cole, L.C. 1952.
"The triangle in child placement: Parent, child and foster parents." *Social Service Review 25: 169–80.*

Comptroller General's Report to the Congress. 1977.
Preventing Mental Retardation—More Can Be Done. Washington, D.C.: U.S. General Accounting Office.

Cook, Timothy. 1983.
"The substantive due process rights of mentally disabled clients." *Mental Disability Law Reporter* 7: 346–57.
Cooke, Robert E. 1969.
"The free choice principle in the care of the mentally retarded." Pp. 361–65 in President's Committee on Mental Retardation, ed., *Changing Patterns in Residential Services for the Mentally Retarded*. Washington, D.C.: U.S. Department of Health, Education, and Welfare.
Copeland, William C., and Iver A. Iversen. 1980a.
"Medicaid Funding for the Continuum of Care for MR/DD Persons: A Policy Memo." Minneapolis: University of Minnesota. Mimeo.
1980b. "Not Just the Aged, Not Just Health Care, and Not Just Nursing Homes." Minneapolis: University of Minnesota. Mimeo.
Corwin, R.B. 1961.
"Role conceptions and career aspirations: A study of identity in nursing." *Sociological Quarterly* 2: 69–86.
Coser, R. L. 1966.
"Role distance, sociological ambivalence and transitional status systems." *American Journal of Sociology* 72: 173–87.
Council for Exceptional Children. 1981.
"Second P.L. 94-142 report sent to lawmakers." *Insights* 12: 1–6.
Darlington, Richard B., Jacqueline M. Royce, Ann Stanton Snipper, Harry W. Murray, and Irving Lazar. 1980.
"Preschool programs and later school competence of children from low-income families." *Science* 208: 202–4.
Davids, L. 1968.
"The Foster Father Role." Ph.D dissertation, New York University.
de Salva, R.M. and P. Fuflak. 1976.
"From institution to community." *Mental Retardation*. 14: 25–28.
"The developmental model: Seeks the positive." 1979.
Mental Retardation News 28: 4–6.
Douglas, Jack D., ed. 1970.
Deviance and Respectability: The Social Construction of Moral Meanings. New York: Basic Books.
Duffy, Frank. 1982.
"Topical display of evoked potentials: Clinical application of brain electrical mapping (BEAM)." *Annals, New York Academy of Sciences* 388: 183–96.
Edgerton, R.B. 1967.
The Cloak of Competence: Stigma in the Lives of the Mentally Retarded. Berkeley: University of California Press.
Edgerton, R.B. and S.M. Bercovici. 1976.
"The cloak of competence: Years later." *American Journal of Mental Deficiency* 80: 485–97.
Fanshel, David. 1966.
Foster Parenthood: A Role Analysis. Minneapolis: University of Minnesota Press.
Fanshel, David, and Eugene B. Shinn. 1978.
Children in Foster Care: A Longitudinal Investigation. New York: Columbia University Press.
Fellener, I.W. and C. Solomon. 1973.
"Achieving permanent solutions for children in foster home care." *Child Welfare* 52: 178–87.

Fisher, Delbert A., et al. 1979.
"Screening for congenital hypothyroidism: Results of screening of one million North American infants." *Journal of Pediatrics* 94: 700–705.
Flanagan, Patrick. 1980.
Proceedings of the conference "Future Directions for the 80's: Ensuring the Viability and Comprehensiveness of Community Service for Mentally Retarded and other Developmentally Disabled Persons." Madison, Wis. 28–30 September 1980. University of Wisconsin Rehabilitation Research and Training Center in Mental Retardation.
Fox, Alice M., and Maurice L. Druzin. 1983.
"Biophysical tests of fetal well being." *Pediatric Annals* 12: 120–31.
Galaway, B. 1972.
"Clarifying the role of foster parents." *Children Today* 1: 32–33.
Garrett, B. 1970.
"Foster family services for mentally retarded children." *Children* 17: 228–33.
Geiser, Robert. 1973.
The Illusion of Caring: Children in Foster Care. Boston: Beacon Press.
Gettings, Robert M. 1980.
Utilization of the Federal/State Medical Assistance Program on Behalf of the Mentally Retarded Persons: A Discussion of Relevant Federal Policy Issues. National Association of State Mental Retardation Program Directors. Mimeo.
Glasser, Ira. 1978.
"Prisoners of Benevolence: Power Versus Liberty in the Welfare State." Pp. 99-168 in *Doing Good—The Limits of Benevolence.* New York: Pantheon Books
Goffman, Erving. 1959.
The Presentation of Self in Everyday Life. New York: Doubleday.
1963. *Stigma: Notes on the Management of Spoiled Identity.* Englewood Cliffs, N.J.: Prentice-Hall.
Gold, Raymond L. 1964.
"In the Basement—The Apartment-building janitor." Pp. 1–49 in Peter L. Berger, ed., *The Human Shape of Work.* New York: Crowell, Collier, and Macmillan.
Gottesfeld, Harry. 1970.
In Loco Parentis: A Study of the Perceived Role Values in Foster Home Care. New York: Jewish Child Care Association of America.
Grunewald, K. 1979.
"Mentally retarded children and young people in Sweden." *Acta Paediatr. Scand.* Suppl. 275: 75–84.
Haitch, Richard. 1968.
Orphans of the Living: The Foster Care Crisis. New York: Public Affairs Commission.
Hansen, Holger. 1978.
"Prevention and liberalized abortion." *American Journal of Mental Deficiency* 83: 185–88.
Hogan, M.F. 1980.
"Normalization and communication: Implementation of a regional community-integrated service system." Pp. 299–312 in R.J. Flynn and K.E. Nitsch, eds., *Normalization, Social Integration, and Community Services.* Baltimore: University Park Press.
Hull, John T. and Joy C. Thompson. 1980.
"Predicting adaptive functioning of mentally retarded persons in community settings." *American Journal of Mental Deficiency* 83: 253–61.

Huntington, Mary Jean. 1957.
"The Development of a Professional Self-Image." Pp. 179–87 in Robert K. Merton, George C. Reader, and Patricia L. Kendall, eds., *The Student-Physician.* Cambridge: Harvard University Press.

Intagliata, James, Sharon Kraus, and Barry Willer. 1980.
"The impact of deinstitutionalization on a community based service system." *Mental Retardation* 18: 305–7.

Jacobs, Dorothy. 1980.
"Foster Care: Myths and Realities." Pp. 89–103 in Herbert Cohen and David Kligler, eds., *Urban Community Care for the Developmentally Disabled.* Springfield, Ill.: Charles Thomas.

Janicki, Matthew P., Tadashii: Mayeda, and William A. Epple. 1983.
"Availability of group homes for persons with mental retardation in the United States." *Mental Retardation* 21, no. 2: 45–51.

Jenkins, Shirley, and Elaine Norman. 1972.
Filial Deprivation and Foster Care. New York: Columbia University Press.

Kadushin, Alfred. 1971.
"Child Welfare: Adoption and Foster Care." Pp. 103–11 in *Encyclopedia of Social Work*, Vol. 1. New York: National Association of Social Workers.

Kadushin, C. 1969.
"The professional self-concept of music students." *American Journal of Sociology* 75: 389–404.

Kolata, Gina. 1983.
"Brain-grafting work shows promise." *Science* 221: 1277.

Lakin, K. Charlie. 1983.
"New admissions and readmissions to a national sample of public residential facilities." *American Journal of Mental Deficiency.* 88: 13–20.

Lakin, K. Charlie, and Robert H. Bruininks. 1980.
Personnel Management and Quality of Residential Services for Developmentally Disabled People. Minneapolis: University of Minnesota.

Landesman-Dwyer, Sharon. 1981.
Living in the Community. Seattle: University of Washington.

Landesman-Dwyer, Sharon, Gerson Berkson, and Daniel Romer. 1979.
"Affiliation and friendship of mentally retarded residents in group homes." *American Journal of Mental Deficiency* 83: 571–79.

Landesman-Dwyer, Sharon, Gene P. Sackett, and Jody Stein Kleinman. 1984.
"Small community residence: The relationship of size to resident and staff behavior." *American Journal of Mental Deficiency* (in press).

Landesman-Dwyer, Sharon, Judith J. Schuckit, and L. Susanne Keller. 1976.
Survey of Developmentally Disabled Clients in Nursing Homes and Congregate Care Facilities. Olympia, Wash.: Department of Social Research and Health Services Planning and Research Division.

Landesman-Dwyer, Sharon, Jody G. Stein, and Gene P. Sackett. 1976
Group Homes for the Mentally Retarded: An Ecological and Behavioral Study. Olympia, Wash.: Department of Social and Health Services Planning and Research Division.

Landesman-Dwyer, Sharon, and Frederica MacL. Sulzbacher.
"Residential Placement and Adaptation of Severely and Profoundly Retarded Individuals." In R. Bruininks, ed., American Association on Mental Deficiency. Monograph No. 4 (in press).

Lewin and Associates. 1979.
   Deinstitutionalization of Mentally Retarded and Other Developmentally Disabled Persons: Lessons from the Experience of Five States. Washington, D.C.: Lewin and Associates.
McCoy, J. 1962a.
   "The application of the role concept of foster parenthood." *Social Casework* 43: 252–56.
1962b. "The motives and conflicts in foster parenthood." *Children* 9: 222–26.
MacEachron, Ann E. 1983.
   "Institutional reform and adaptive functioning of mentally retarded persons: A field experiment." *American Journal of Mental Deficiency* 88, no. 1: 2–12.
Magrab, Phyllis. 1981.
   Community Workbook for Collaborative Service to Preschool Handicapped Children. Washington, D.C.: American Association of University Affiliated Programs.
Marcus, Steven. 1978.
   "Their brothers' keeper: An episode from English history." Pp. 41-66 in *Doing Good–The Limits of Benevolence.* New York: Pantheon Books.
Merton, Robert K. 1968.
   "Continuities in the theory of reference groups and social structure." Pp. 335–440 in *Social Theory and Social Structure.* 2nd ed. New York: Free Press.
Nadler, Henry L. 1976.
   "Prenatal detection of genetic defects." *Advances in Pediatrics* 22: 1–81.
National Council on the Handicapped. 1983.
   Annual Report, March 1983, Washington, D.C.
National Institute of Child Health and Human Development. 1979.
   Analysis of Research Supported by the Center for Research for Mothers and Children: Fiscal Years 1970–1978. Washington, D.C.: National Institute of Child Health and Human Development.
National Study Group on State Medicaid Strategies. 1983.
   Restructuring Medicaid: An Agenda for Change. Summary Report of the National Study Group on State Medicaid Strategies. Washington, D.C.: The Center for the Study of Social Policy.
Neal, David, and David L. Kirp. 1983.
   The Allure of Legalization Reconsidered: The Case of Special Education. Rpt. no. 82-A27. Stanford University: School of Education Institute for Research on Educational Finance and Governance Project.
Nelson, Stanley M. 1980.
   Program Models and Service Configurations. A paper presented at the Conference on Ensuring the Viability and Comprehensiveness of Community Services for the Mentally Retarded and Other Developmentally Disabled Persons. Madison, Wis.
New York State Commission on Quality of Care for the Mentally Disabled. 1980.
   Willowbrook: From Institution to Community. A Fiscal and Programmatic Review of Selected Community Residences in New York City. Albany.
Office of Employee Services. 1979.
   Final Report of the Office of Employee Services. Philadelphia: Human Services Associates.
Office of the Inspector General. 1984.
   A Program Inspection on Transition of Developmentally Disabled Young Adults from School to Adult Services. Washington, D.C.: Office of Program Inspections, Office of the Inspector General, Dept. of Health and Human Services.

Office of Technological Assessment, Congress of the United States. 1982.
   Technology and Handicapped People. Washington, D.C.: U.S. Government
   Printing Office.
Ougheltree, Cornelia 1957.
   Finding Foster Homes. New York: Child Welfare League of America.
Pavalko, R.M. 1971.
   "Occupational ideologies." Pp. 192–95 in *Sociology of Occupations and Profes-
   sions.* Itasca, Ill.: Peacock Publishers.
Pollard, Anderson. N.d.
   Inter-Organizational Task Group-Living Environment: An Action Policy Propo-
   sal. President's Committee on Mental Retardation Community Support Services
   and Systems Task Group.
Pratt, Michael W., and Mary A. Luszcz. 1980.
   "Measuring dimension of the quality of care in small residential communities."
   American Journal of Mental Deficiency. 85: 188-94.
President's Committee on Mental Retardation. 1969.
   Changing Patterns in Residential Care for the Mentally Retarded. Washington,
   D.C.: U.S. Government Printing Office.
   1976a. *Changing Patterns in Residential Care for the Mentally Retarded.* Rev. ed.
   Washington, D.C.: U.S. Government Printing Office.
   1976b. *Mental Retardation. Century of Decision.* Washington, D.C.: U.S.
   Government Printing Office.
   1977a. *International Summit on Prevention of Mental Retardation from Biomedical Causes.* Washington, D.C.: U.S. Government Printing Office.
   1977b. *Mental Retardation: Past and Present MR 76.* Washington, D.C.: U.S.
   Government Printing Office.
   1979. *Mental Retardation: The Leading Edge—Service Programs That Work.*
   Washington, D.C.: U.S. Government Printing Office.
   1980a. *Mental Retardation: Prevention Strategies That Work.* Washington, D.C.:
   U.S. Government Printing Office.
   1980b. *New Neighbors: The Retarded Citizen in Quest of a Home.* Washington,
   D.C.: U.S. Government Printing Office.
President's Panel on Mental Retardation. 1962.
   *A Proposal for National Actions to Combat Mental Retardation: Report to the
   President.* Washington, D.C.: U.S. Government Printing Office.
Purpura, Dominick P., James J. Gallagher, and Theodore D. Tjossem. 1980.
   Mental Retardation Research: A Five Year Program. New York: Kennedy
   Center, Albert Einstein College of Medicine.
Pykett, Ian L. 1983.
   "NMR imaging in medicine." *Scientific American* 246 no. 5: 78–88.
Raynes, N.V., N.M. Pratt, and S. Roses. 1977.
   "Aides' involvement in decision-making and the quality of care in institutional
   settings." *American Journal of Mental Deficiency* 81: 570–77.
Reistroffer, M. 1968.
   "A university extension course for foster parents." *Children* 15: 28–31.
Reiter, Shemit, and A.M. Levi. 1980.
   "Factors affecting social integration of noninstitutionalized mentally retarded
   adults." *American Journal of Mental Deficiency* 85: 25–30.
Rotegard, L.L., B.K. Hill, and R.H. Bruininks. 1983.
   "Environmental characteristics of residential facilities for mentally retarded per-
   sons in the United States." *American Journal of Mental Deficiency* 88, no. 1: 49–56.

Rowitz, Louis 1980a.
"Original identifiers of mental retardation in a clinic population." *American Journal of Mental Deficiency* 85: 82–86.
1980b. Professionalism, Manpower Development and Mental Disability: Conflict and Resolution. Paper presented at 1st Annual Fogarty Memorial Conference: Changing Governmental Policies for the Mentally Disabled. Newport, R.I.

Sagarin, Edward. 1975.
Deviants and Deviance: An Introduction to the Study of Disvalued People and Behavior. New York: Praeger.

Sarason, Seymour. 1966.
"Forward." In Bert Blatt, *Christmas in Purgatory: A Photographic Essay.* Boston: Allyn and Bacon.

Sarbin, Theodore R., and Vernon l. Allen. 1968.
"Role theory." Pp. 488–567 in Gardner Lindzey and Elliot Aranson, eds., *The Handbook of Social Psychology*, Vol. 1. Reading, Mass.: Addison-Wesley.

Schalock, Robert S., and Roger S. Harper. 1978.
"Placement from community-based mental retardation programs: How well do clients do?" *American Journal of Mental Deficiency* 83: 240-47.

Scheerenberger, Richard C. 1979.
Public Residential Services for the Mentally Retarded. Madison, Wis.: National Association of Superintendents of Public Residential Facilities.
1980. *Community Program and Services.* Madison, Wis.: National Association of Superintendents of Public Residential Facilities.
N.d. Human service person power for developmentally disabled persons.

Schneider, Morton. 1983.
"Neonatal cranial ultrasound." *Pediatric Annals* 12: 133–39.

Shapiro, Deborah. 1976.
Agencies and Foster Children. New York: Columbia University Press.

Simpson, Ida Harper. 1979.
From Student to Nurse: A Longitudinal Study of Socialization. Cambridge: Harvard University Press.

Simpson, R. L., and I. H. Simpson. 1959.
"The psychiatric attendant: Development of an occupational self-image in a low-status occupation." *American Sociological Review* 24: 389–92.

Sitkei, C. George. 1980.
"After group home living– What alternatives? Results of a two year mobility followup study." *Mental Retardation* 1:9–13.

Smith, Francis W. 1983.
"NMR imaging in pediatric practice." *Pediatrics* 71: 852–54.

Sokoloff, H. David. 1980a.
Address to A.A.M.D. Regional Conference.
1980b. Presentation to the California State Developmental Disabilities Council. San Francisco: Adult Services Committee.

Sokolovsky, J., C. Cohen, D. Berger, and J. Geiger. 1978.
"Personal networks of ex-mental patients in a Manhattan SRO hotel." *Human Organization* 37: 5–15.

Stack, C. 1974.
All Our Kin: Strategies of Survival in a Black Community. New York: Harper & Row.

Stacy, Donald, Daniel M. Doleys, and Roger Malcolm. 1979.
   "Effects of social skills training in a community-based program." American
   Journal of Mental Deficiency 84: 152–58.
Stein, Theodore, Eileen Gambrill, and Kermit Wiltse. 1978.
   Children in Foster Homes: Achieving Continuity of Care. New York: Praeger.
Suttes, Patricia. 1980.
   "Environmental variables related to community placement failure in mentally
   retarded adults." *Mental Retardation* 18: 189–91.
Suttes, Patricia, Tadashi Mayeda, and Tom Call. 1980.
   "Comparison of successfully and unsuccessfully community placed mentally
   retarded persons." *American Journal of Mental Deficiency* 85: 262–67.
Swindall, B. E. 1961.
   "The function and role of the natural parent in the foster family constellation."
   Child Welfare 40: 6–11.
Thomas, L. 1971.
   "The technology of medicine." *New England Journal of Medicine* 285, no. 24
   (Dec. 9): 1366–68.
Todd, Seldon P., Jr., and Michael Greelis. 1981.
   National Networking: A Case Study. Menlo Park, Calif.: American Association
   of University Affiliated Programs and The Institute for the Future.
Townsend, P. 1957.
   The Family Life of Older People. London: Routledge & Kegan Paul.
Treudley, M. B. 1944.
   "The concept of role in social work." *American Sociological Review* 9: 665–70.
U.S. Department of Education. 1984.
   *To Assure the Free and Appropriate Education of All Handicapped Children:
   Sixth Annual Report on the Implementation of P.L. 94-142. The Education for All
   Handicapped Children's Act.* Washington, D.C.: U.S. Government Printing
   Office.
U.S. Office of Education. 1979a.
   Progress Toward a Free Appropriate Public Education. Washington, D.C.: U.S.
   Government Printing Office.
   1979b. *Lasting Effects After Preschool.* Washington, D.C.: U.S. Government
      Printing Office.
U.S. Department of Health, Education and Welfare. 1977.
   *Federal Research Activity in Mental Retardation: A Review with Recom-
   mendations for the Future.* Washington, D.C.: U.S. Government Printing Office.
Urban Institute. 1979.
   *Alternative Community Living Arrangement and Non-Vocational Social Develop-
   ment Service—State of the Art.* Washington, D.C.: The Urban Institute.
Vick, J. 1967.
   "Recruiting and retaining foster homes." *Public Welfare* 25: 229–34.
Wardwall, W. I. 1955.
   "The reduction of strain in a marginal social role." *American Journal of Sociology*
   61: 16–25.
Weinstein, Eugene. 1960.
   The Self-Image of the Foster Child. New York: Russell Sage.
Whitehead, Claude W. 1979.
   "Sheltered workshops in the decade ahead: Work and wages, or welfare."
   P. 73 in G. Thomas Bellamy, Gail O'Connor, and Orv C. Karah, eds., *Vocational*

Rehabilitation of Severely Handicapped Persons: Contemporary Service Strategies. Baltimore: University Park Press.

Wieck, Colleen, and Robert H. Bruininks. 1980.
The Cost of Public and Community Residential Care for Mentally Retarded People in the United States. Project Rpt. No. 9. Minneapolis: University of Minnesota Developmental Disability Project on Residential Service and Community Adjustment.

Wiegerink, Ronald, and John W. Pelosi. 1979.
Developmental Disabilities: The D.D. Movement. Baltimore: Paul H. Brookes, Publishers.

Wilkes, J.R. 1974.
"The impact of fostering on the fostering family." *Child Welfare* 53: 373–79.

Williston, G.C. 1963.
"The foster-parent role." *Journal of Social Psychology* 60: 263–72.

Wilsnack, William. 1980.
Living Environment for the Mentally Retarded: An Action Policy Proposal. Washington, D.C.: President's Committee on Mental Retardation.

Wolfensberger, Wolf. 1972.
The Principle of Normalization in Human Services. Toronto: National Institute on Mental Retardation.

Wolins, Martin. 1963.
Selecting Foster Parents: The Ideal and the Reality. New York: Columbia University Press.

Zigler, Edward. 1978.
"National crisis in mental retardation." *American Journal of Mental Deficiency* 83: 1–8.

INDEX